I0819367

ADVANCE PRAISE FOR *IN FERTILITY*

"A remarkable story that will resonate with so many readers on their own journeys in fertility."

—Leah Hazard, bestselling author of *Womb: The Inside Story of Where We All Began*

"The ideal way to create a book about the terrifying ups and downs of in vitro fertilization would be to assign an award-winning investigative journalist and writer to go through the soul-shaking process over and over and over again, with every conceivable outcome, and then have her write about it. Though it wasn't designed that way, *In Fertility* is that book. An engrossing, profoundly personal and yet crisply objective journey through the harrowing, ever-so-human wilderness of in vitro fertilization and the business of laboratory conception."

—Ian Brown, award-winning author of *The Boy in the Moon* and *Sixty*

"*In Fertility* is both memoir and exposé, but it reads like a page-turner. Kathryn Blaze Baum brings her seasoned journalist's unflinching eye to an industry where costs and stakes run sky-high—and business is conducted inside women's bodies, including the author's own. *In Fertility* illuminates a subject of intimate importance to millions of Canadians, and makes visible the suffering that is too often invisible. It is also a gripping story, movingly told."

—Emma Knight, Giller-shortlisted author of *The Life Cycle of the Common Octopus*

"Anyone considering fertility treatments should first read this book. *In Fertility* is a no-holds-barred examination of the labyrinthine process, the medical minutiae, the multi-billion-dollar baby-making industry and the punishing costs (physical, emotional and financial), combined with Kathryn Blaze Baum's deeply personal reflections on the life-altering impacts of IVF and surrogacy."

—André Picard, award-winning health reporter and bestselling author of *Neglected No More*

"*In Fertility* is a powerful, deeply needed guide for anyone struggling to get pregnant. It's also an invaluable resource for the people in their lives who are supporting them. I wish I had had something like this when so many of my friends were in the trenches. The book is part impeccably reported science journalism, part memoir, and at times reads almost like a thriller."

—Robyn Doolittle, award-winning journalist and bestselling author of *Had It Coming*

"Kathryn Blaze Baum's *In Fertility* is a must-read for anyone embarking on the uncertain journey of starting or growing a family. Baum does for infertility what Emily Oster did for pregnancy—this is both a riveting personal account that is candid and thoughtful, and a highly informative and balanced exploration of an industry and process that touches so many, yet few know the truth about. I'm so grateful this book exists, and for Baum's brave and compassionate voice."

—Ashley Audrain, bestselling author of *The Push* and *The Whispers*

"Kathryn Blaze Baum expertly weaves her deeply personal fertility saga with an incisive investigation of the fertility industry and a thoughtful exploration of the ethics of surrogacy. The result is a brave, vulnerable and unflinchingly honest book that will be a source of wisdom and solace for countless people on their journeys to parenthood."

—Alexandra Posadzki, award-winning author of *Rogers v. Rogers: The Battle for Control of Canada's Telecom Empire*

"A deeply informative indictment of our baby-mad culture that blames people with uteruses for their failure—and, yes, we treat it as failure—to bear children, and then fails *them* medically, financially, logistically and informationally when they seek help."

—Anna Mehler Paperny, bestselling author of *Hello I Want to Die Please Fix Me*

IN FERTILITY

The Story of a Miracle and the Big Business Behind It

KATHRYN BLAZE BAUM

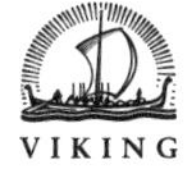

VIKING

VIKING
an imprint of Penguin Canada,
a division of Penguin Random House Canada Limited

Canada • USA • UK • Ireland • Australia • New Zealand •
India • South Africa • China

First published 2026

Viking, an imprint of Penguin Canada
A division of Penguin Random House Canada
320 Front Street West, Suite 1400
Toronto, Ontario, M5V 3B6, Canada
penguinrandomhouse.ca

The authorized representative in the EU for product safety and compliance is Penguin Random House Ireland, Morrison Chambers, 32 Nassau Street, Dublin D02 YH68, Ireland, https://eu-contact.penguin.ie

LIBRARY AND ARCHIVES CANADA CATALOGUING IN PUBLICATION

Title: In fertility : the story of a miracle and the big business behind it / Kathryn Blaze Baum.
Names: Baum, Kathryn Blaze, author.
Description: Includes index.
Identifiers: Canadiana (print) 20250245167 | Canadiana (ebook) 20250249073 | ISBN 9780735249592 (hardcover) | ISBN 9780735249608 (EPUB)
Subjects: LCSH: Baum, Kathryn Blaze—Health. | LCSH: Infertility, Female—Patients—Canada—Biography. |LCSH: Journalists—Canada—Biography. | LCSH: Infertility—Treatment—Canada. | LCSH: Human reproductive technology—Canada. | LCGFT: Autobiographies.
Classification: LCC RG201 .B53 2026 | DDC 362.1981780092—dc23

Book design by Lisa Jager
Typeset by Terra Page and Six Red Marbles
Cover design by Lisa Jager

Printed in Canada

10 9 8 7 6 5 4 3 2 1

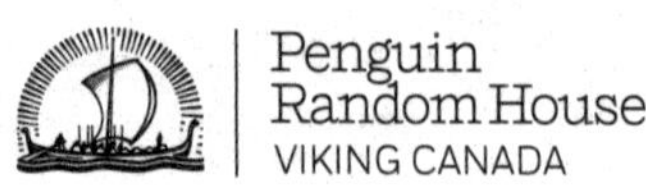

FOR

KENDRA AND STACEY

"A wounded deer leaps highest."

—EMILY DICKINSON

CONTENTS

INTRODUCTION

Great Expectations

THERE'S A SMALL linen box in my closet, hidden behind a stack of sweaters. I tucked it there so I could honour its contents without having to constantly face its existence. The beige lid is embossed with numbers in gold foil: *09.04.2019.*

April was when I had the miscarriage that started it all, the first of several in the odyssey my husband, Dan, and I embarked on to create a sibling for our daughter, Sidney, who was naturally conceived and born the year before. My close friends gave me the keepsake box to store the sonogram of the baby that never made its way earthside. They knew it would be gut-wrenching to throw out the image but also heartbreaking to do anything with it other than set it aside.

Over time, the box became a mausoleum of losses. One after another, I added black-and-white sonograms of near-life that, for one reason or another, some known and some unknown, never became much more than they were in those hauntingly sweet images. We had turned to in vitro fertilization (IVF) to help grow our family, but even assisted reproductive technologies couldn't protect us from the heartbreak of miscarriage, from all the uncertainty that comes with struggling to make a baby. There's only so much that science can tell us about infertility. To be the subject of so many unanswered questions was a kind of torture that only the most sadistic of fiction writers could conjure.

Infertility is typically thought of as a failure to achieve a pregnancy after twelve or more months of regular, unprotected sex. By that definition, I wasn't infertile. *Getting* pregnant wasn't my problem. It was *staying* pregnant. A broader diagnosis of infertility encompasses cases like mine, defining the disease as the inability to achieve a successful pregnancy.

As our treatment saga wore on, with every poke and probe and appointment at the fertility clinic, I became ever more committed to one day telling our story. I'm an investigative reporter with *The Globe and Mail*, Canada's national newspaper. It's my job to ask questions and write stories. I have reported on justice, politics, crime, health, education, Indigenous issues, religion, business, climate change and public policy. I have covered terrorist attacks, natural disasters, mass shootings and historic elections in Canada and the United States. I've been working as a reporter since 2008. It's hard to take off the journalist hat and not see the world from that perspective.

I would lie on the clinic exam table, feet in stirrups, staring up at the ceiling, and think to myself, "One day I will write about all this." I wanted to write the book I wish I'd read while we were trying to grow our family. I wanted to explore the mysterious, deeply interesting aspects of fertility treatment in a way that combined our personal narrative with research and interviews with doctors, patients, lawyers, surrogates, scientists, business owners, policymakers and academics. I wanted to help people navigate the labyrinthine process and arm them with information so they could go into treatment as clear-eyed as possible. I wanted to offer fertility patients and their loved ones comfort and support through storytelling; I wanted to help them handle the emotional toll of loss and yearning. And I wanted to give people an unvarnished sense of what IVF entails so they could protect their hearts and bodies. The result is a book that blends memoir and in-depth reporting.

My experience touched myriad aspects of treatment, but of course not all of them. There are so many paths that a fertility journey can take. I had to put up guardrails on the scope of my book, else the research, interview and writing process would have become entirely unwieldy. My journey didn't include, for example, the selection and use of donor eggs or donor sperm, so I don't delve deeply into the issues and emotions around that. I should also note that it's not the norm for a journey to be as intractable as mine was—some people move through treatment with relative ease, in a straight line, with positive results at every juncture—but my experience is, overall, representative and illustrative.

Although my story is unique because it's mine, it is, at its core, all too common. One in six people globally struggles with infertility, and it will only get worse because of social and environmental factors, such as the decision to have children later in life, the rising rate of obesity and increased exposure to endocrine-disrupting chemicals. An estimated one in five women experiences miscarriage, though the number is thought to be higher given that some losses, particularly very early ones, go unreported or even undetected. Sperm counts and sperm quality are on the decline.

Infertility can arise for any number of reasons, including irregular or absent ovulation, blocked fallopian tubes, hormone issues, structural problems with the uterus or issues with sperm. I confronted what's known as secondary infertility, which is the inability to get pregnant or carry a pregnancy to term after previously giving birth.

Like primary infertility, its rates are rising. A lot of the underlying emotions, treatments and feelings of isolation are shared. If you've had one child and you're struggling to make another, all the optimism you hear, especially from doctors, can be frustrating. *You've done it before, so you'll do it again.* A lot can change from one pregnancy or birth to the next. I know this first-hand. It's hard to be reassured.

If you're several years into your quest to have your first child, I wouldn't blame you for bristling at the very premise of this book—my journey, for that matter. I wouldn't blame you for calling me greedy for wanting more than the one child I already had, for feeling that I might never understand your specific pain. While I did experience a pregnancy loss before conceiving Sid, I do not know the hell of going through my child-bearing years wondering *if* I will ever become a mother.

It's not a misery competition. It's not about who has it worse, who is more of a wounded warrior. The compassion I feel for people trying to claw their way to their first child could not be more deeply felt. If you are one of these people, I'm lending you my hope. It's not fair.

Until a few short decades ago, people struggling with infertility could turn only to less invasive treatments that worked in certain narrow circumstances. If those approaches weren't successful, there was no path to a biological child. Once experimental, IVF has become relatively mainstream in developed countries among those who can afford it. IVF as we know it today involves a retrieval, in which eggs are extracted from ovaries; fertilization, in which eggs are fertilized by sperm in a lab; and an embryo transfer, in which a fresh or frozen embryo is placed into a uterus in the hopes that it will implant and develop into a baby.

In 2025, a single IVF cycle typically cost around $20,000 in Canada or the United States, give or take several thousands of dollars depending on the drug protocol and any add-on treatments. Most patients have to do more than one cycle before a successful pregnancy. No one is guaranteed a baby, though some clinics now offer services at a bloated cost with a baby-or-your-money-back guarantee. Surrogacy, when needed, adds further expense with costs ranging from tens of thousands of dollars, in cases where surrogates are reimbursed for their expenses but not compensated, to upward of a half-million dollars in the United States in situations involving agencies that provide "express" matching services for a salaried surrogacy journey.

The big business of fertility is booming. The global fertility services market was valued at over US$21 billion in 2021 and is projected to more than quadruple by 2031. There are incredible tailwinds in the space: the trend of delayed child-bearing and the associated increased infertility rates; a rise in non-heterosexual people seeking to start or grow their families; the evolving technology; the high margins. Advanced female age and diminished egg reserve are among the top reasons for seeking treatment, behind sperm issues and unexplained infertility, which is a condition whereby standard fertility testing fails to explain why a person or couple can't get or stay pregnant.

The concept of the "ticking biological clock" is, unfortunately, well-founded. Miscarriage rates increase with age, and IVF success rates decrease. This is why more and more people are choosing to preserve their eggs in a process that's been dubbed social egg freezing. (This is in contrast to medical egg freezing, which is done for health reasons, for example in advance of cancer treatments that may damage reproductive organs.)

It's a matter of debate whether the rise of social egg freezing is a good thing. On one hand, it allows a person to take some measure of control over their fertility, providing at least a modicum of comfort that their younger eggs will be there for them in the future. On the other hand, that sense of comfort can be false and comes at great physical and financial expense. The reality is that after spending thousands of dollars freezing their eggs, most people don't go back for them later.

Several people I spoke with for this book said they prioritized their career over starting a family. "I really liked what I was doing, work-wise," one woman told me. "I would think, 'I'll wait six months until this project is over' or 'Once I get through this deadline, we'll start trying.' If I had known then what I know now, I would have said, 'Screw the project. Screw the deadline.'" All of them said they wished they had been better informed, at an earlier age, about the correlation between aging and infertility.

Few minds are noisier than that of a person going through IVF. The journey, by its very nature, is all consuming. It takes over your days, spent at the clinic or waiting by the phone or computer for test results and medication instructions. It takes over your body, hormonally and physically. It should come as no surprise that it takes over your mind.

"The pressure squeezes you," one woman living in the United Kingdom and struggling with infertility told me. "Whether it's financial pressure, the ticking-clock pressure, the sibling-age-gap pressure. It squeezes you and squeezes you."

Dan and I are privileged to have had the financial means to not only start IVF but to keep going and going and going and going. So many people are unable to do so. Infertility—and the pressure it creates—doesn't discriminate between the rich and poor. And the disparity in access to treatment is vast. If you've got time and money, you'll probably be able to have a baby if you persist. One day, one way. That's the sad reality.

You might think that because I eventually came out the other side with a bigger family that I will be evangelical about IVF, that

I will sing the praises of the baby-making industry and laud it as a panacea. But I'm not. And I won't. That wouldn't be my honest truth, and it wouldn't honour or reflect the experiences of the people I interviewed. It's not uncommon for patients to end up resenting their doctors and harbouring ill feelings toward their clinics, especially if those doctors and clinics didn't end up making them a baby. It's to be expected that a patient's memories of their journey will be far from fond, even in the best of circumstances.

There are aspects of the IVF process in Canada I believe must be improved, particularly as it relates to protecting the consumer—that is, the patient. The federal government appears to have thrown its hands up after a Supreme Court ruling neutered large parts of the act that governs reproductive medicine. Access to care and funding varies wildly depending on a patient's postal code. There are some provinces and territories that don't have a single IVF clinic. Accountability is lacking. Clinics aren't required to publish their success rates. There are no national, standardized criteria for disclosing IVF complications. There's no system for regulating or licensing embryologists. There's no licensing regime for surrogacy agencies, and the way some of them operate might even be illegal under federal law, if only on paper. Clinics push add-on services that cost thousands of dollars and might not improve the chances of conception.

These concerns are not unique to Canada. There are problems with access, funding and transparency in the United States, Europe and beyond. All of the above says nothing of all the ways we're missing the mark in educating young people about their fertility so they can make better decisions about when and how to start their family.

Fertility patients, no matter where they live or seek treatment, are often uninformed and desperate. It's a dangerous combination. Patients are willing to go into debt, take out a second mortgage, sacrifice everything. As one long-time fertility doctor put it to me, there's a "dark side" to the massive and growing industry in which people "prey on their patients' fears."

In doing my reporting for this book, I reopened old wounds. New details were revealed to me, both about our personal case and about the business of conceiving—about the regulatory, medical, ethical, financial and societal forces that underpin the fertility sector in Canada and elsewhere. Some of the conversations I had with patients and experts caused me to think differently about decisions we made with our baby-making blinders on. The more information I got, the more I came to terms with the reality that fertility treatment is an exercise in sliding doors. Had we done one thing differently, our entire journey might have been changed. Complex cases in particular don't follow a neat and tidy decision-tree. *If this happens, do that. If that happens, do this.* Fertility care is not that straightforward. What works in one instance might not work in another, sometimes for good reason and sometimes for no good reason at all.

This book, then, isn't about the outcome. It's about the effort, the journey, the messy middle. It's about the village that brought our children to us—the total strangers who impacted our lives in ways they can't possibly fully understand. They taught us what it means to be brave and selfless. They made their way to us when we were at our most broken, restoring our faith in our dream and in humanity.

The measure of a successful or "good" fertility story isn't just whether you end up with a baby. That shouldn't be the sole metric. You can have a horrible experience *and* come out of it with a child. The two are not mutually exclusive. I still have flashbacks and can well up on a dime. That's why the linen box is tucked away in my closet, hidden but still there. The losses are in the past; they led to my present and will be ever with me in the future. They're part of me.

I'm not particularly religious or spiritual, but I have chosen to think of those lost souls as our family's angels. There were certainly times over the course of our treatment that I wished I was devoutly religious. Dan and I are Jewish, mostly by manner of tradition, ritual and identity. I don't believe in a higher being the way you do if you're somebody who says things like "Give it up to God," "God doesn't make mistakes" or "God has a plan."

What got me through the quest wasn't a belief in God. It wasn't my belief in fate. It was my belief in free will. It was my belief in my power to control my emotions when I couldn't control anything else. When I was at rock bottom, I made a promise to myself: I wouldn't let our dream of a bigger family swallow what Dan and I already had—a daughter who deserved for us to be present and really truly *with her*; our health; and each other, a love for the ages.

When we were at our lowest, someone who overcame infertility told Dan and me to be "open to a total fucking miracle." I remember being deeply annoyed. *Easy for her to say.* She was out the other side. She already had her baby. I was all but done with hoping, all but resigned to the notion that it was over for us. I couldn't have known it at the time, but her words were prescient. After all, our quest culminated in an unbelievable plot twist that can only be described as a total fucking miracle.

October 12, 2021

WHEN I OPEN my eyes on October 12, 2021, the perspective is all wrong. I'm lying face down on the floor. Where am I? I press myself up onto an elbow and lift my head. It's dark, but I can see blood dripping from my face. The floor is cold against my naked body.

My brain is trying to make sense of what's happening. *Did someone break into our house? Was I attacked? Where is our three-year-old daughter, Sidney? Is she okay?* I think these things but can't seem to say them. My words are stuck in my throat. My whole body is shaking. My hands are tingling, then numb. A wave of nausea hits me with such force it almost distracts from the pain.

I touch my face. There's a hole where part of my bottom lip should be. Someone has their hands around my waist, trying to roll me over onto my back. I cry out in agony and wriggle free. It feels like daggers are stabbing my ovaries. My insides are on fire. I curl up into the fetal position, terrified, and lock eyes with Dan. His face and voice start to come into focus. He's kneeling beside me, ashen as he tries to calm me down, calm himself down: "It's okay. You're okay. It's okay. You're okay. You're on the bathroom floor. I think you fainted." It's the middle of the night, he explains.

A loud thud had woken him up. He turned over in bed and realized I wasn't beside him. He went into the bathroom and found me there.

I'm near the toilet. Convenient. Bile erupts into the bowl, the foamy yellowish liquid mixing with the blood spilling off my chin. "Call 911," I say through tears as I continue to vomit and shake. It's 2:47 a.m. when Dan places the call.

The paramedics arrive at 2:52 a.m. There are two of them, both men. They're calm, kind, reassuring. I have stopped vomiting, but I'm still on the floor, too weak and in shock to get up. Dan takes a bathrobe and drapes it over me.

"Can you tell us what happened?" one of the paramedics asks, standing over me in the doorway of the bathroom. Dan explains that I was on a bunch of fertility medications for an IVF egg retrieval. I'd never fainted from the drugs before, but I had told Dan several times over the course of the injections that the meds sometimes made me feel light-headed. Just the day before, I had been standing in the kitchen when my vision became distorted and I felt weak in the knees. A kaleidoscope of black and grey spots multiplied and merged closer and closer until the room faded almost to dark. I managed to lower myself safely to the floor, leaning against the dishwasher until it felt safe to stand back up.

The paramedics are confused. Rightly so. If you haven't been through IVF, you likely don't know much about how it works or the toll it can take on a person's body. They have questions. What kind of medications? What's an egg retrieval? Did the procedure already happen? Was I pregnant? *In the nicest way possible, fuck off.* We do our best to explain what happened. I had been injecting myself daily with drugs that caused me to grow dozens of eggs in the follicles of my ovaries. The day before, a doctor extracted the eggs and then an embryologist combined them with Dan's sperm to make embryos.

My mother-in-law sleeps with her phone on loud "in case someone needs me," she has always said. We need her now. She comes over to be at the house with Sid, who is still sleeping. The paramedics load me onto a stretcher at 3:05 a.m. They roll me into the emergency room on a gurney, the throbbing pain in my mouth worsening as the shock wears off.

I muster the courage to look at my face. Turning my phone's camera on myself, I pull back the pack of gauze I had been holding to my mouth and see that my bottom lip is sliced open in the middle. The moist tissue is severed in the shape of a V that dips below my vermilion border. A couple of my teeth, pink with bloodied saliva, peek through, intact. My eyes are puffy from crying, and there are some splotches of blood on my cheeks, chin and in my hair. While it certainly could have been worse, my reflection scares the shit out of me. This isn't the first time I've been beaten up by IVF. But the bloodied sight of myself is striking for its physical representation of the emotional war I'm fighting.

I want another baby. I *need* another baby. The yearning is primal and relentless. It's consuming. A fertility journey is among the most punishing, consequential quests a human being can endure. The rest of my life has faded into the background, the B plot to this main storyline. I don't remember what it's like to think of other things. I don't remember what it's like to be the me I was before all of this. I'm tired—so tired—but I'm not ready to put down arms.

An ER doctor weaves eleven stitches through the border of my bottom lip and discharges me with instructions to return in a few days to have the wiry black sutures removed. When I'm home and settled, I text some of the people closest to me to let them know what had happened. "It's very painful and was so scary waking up on the floor with blood like that, in pain and not knowing why," I write to my sister-in-law, Eileen. "But I'll be okay—and I'm lucky it wasn't my eyes or a head injury."

Her response hits me like a truck. "For some reason, this makes me so angry," she writes. "Maybe it's easier than sadness? . . . Is it finally over? I trust it is. The signs. I think the message is stop. You've done so much work for this and now you stand back and trust the universe. Cliché? Fuck no. It's wisdom. How's Dan? Has Sidney seen it yet? Is it still painful? . . . When will you travel and take distance from this? I love you girl." She wasn't outright telling me to stop, but she was reminding me I had a choice. She was writing me with a clear head and a clear view of what we'd been through. She was making sure I could see the situation for what it was: a rock bottom.

I lie in bed, in pain but most of all scared. How can I justify putting myself through any more of the physical, emotional and mental torment of a prolonged IVF journey? There's a part of me that wants Dan to make the call and say it's over—that whatever happens next, no matter what, I'm done with the surgeries, injections, ultrasounds, bloodwork, appointments, retrievals, all the poking and prodding. I also know that no one can stop me except myself. There would have been no moral failure in us choosing to "give up." To stop trying. To just stop. And be. Perhaps, in fact, it would have taken more courage to practise that kind of acceptance than to resist it.

"I hear you," I write to Eileen. "The universe is begging me. We'll see what happens—whether I have the courage to listen. Hope I don't have to."

Before

I TOOK A seat at my gate at LaGuardia Airport and unfurled my copy of *The New York Times*. As a twenty-three-year-old journalism student at New York University in 2008, reading the paper had become a ritual, a daily lesson in the skills I was honing. I was Toronto bound for March break and planning to stay with a close friend for a few days and visit some family.

With my hair in a messy bun and sporting leggings and an oversized sweatshirt, I was not on the lookout for a romantic connection. I thumbed my way through the paper to the crossword; I grew up doing them with my parents, the day's puzzle tucked into a clipboard on the kitchen counter for us to collectively chip away at. I was making slow progress when a handsome guy in a suit seated next to me leaned over and gave me the correct answer to one of the clues. "Bold," I thought. "Also, impressive." There are few things more attractive to me than confidence and intelligence. We got to chatting. His name was Dan. He had been in New York for a job interview and was now on his way home. It wasn't long before we realized we had some mutual friends in Toronto. It was a wonder we hadn't met before. We had probably been at some of the same bars and parties.

Dan finagled it so that we could sit together on the plane. "Smooth move," I thought, "turning a flight into a date." Our conversation flowed so naturally and we got along so well that we joked about what we would name our kids one day. We exchanged numbers and made plans to go with some friends to a club downtown a few days later. When we met up, he took my hand and guided me through the sweaty crowd to the bar. He bought me a drink and leaned in for a kiss. I liked the way he took charge, the way he went for what he wanted. I liked the way he held my hand and led me.

We kept in close touch when I returned to New York, messaging nonstop on our BlackBerrys and playing an online version of Scrabble. I would rush back to my dorm room to log on to my computer and see if he had played any letters while I was in class. It was a whirlwind courtship. Dan flew me to Dublin when he was there for work and visited me in New York several times. He was so charming that I told my mom I was pretty certain he had girlfriends in multiple cities.

Neither of us had been looking for a life partner. We were in our early twenties and still figuring out who we were. We both knew, though, that we weren't prepared to walk away from each other just because of distance or timing. We understood how rare it is to find someone who can give you butterflies and at the same time make you feel safe.

Still, it took him nearly seven years to propose to me. That wasn't out of character to those who know him well. Dan takes his time deliberating big decisions. By the time we got engaged, we had spent several years doing long distance, one or the other of us in New York, Toronto, Boston or Ottawa. Distance didn't break us, but it did test us. We nearly ended things when he was at business school in Boston and I was in Toronto, working as a reporter at the *Globe*. But we fought our way through and emerged stronger for it. At one point, he told me he felt as if we could "run through walls together." The phrase stuck with me. It became a relationship mantra. We would need it.

Dan hadn't been back from Boston for more than a couple months when my editor asked if I would move to Ottawa for a one-year posting as a political reporter on Parliament Hill. It was a good opportunity. Also, cruel timing. I had for years taken every assignment that was asked of me. Free of any real responsibilities, I had travelled last minute to Haiti in the immediate aftermath of the 2010 earthquake, to Boston to report on the 2013 marathon bombing and ensuing manhunt, to Moncton to cover a string of shootings that killed three Royal Canadian Mounted Police officers in 2014, to remote First Nations reserves to cover murders and social injustices. I wasn't ready to start saying no.

But in saying yes to my career, I knew I was saying "please hold" to my personal life. I knew the move would delay a proposal and marriage and, in turn, starting a family.

I had been on birth control since I was a sixteen-year-old kid growing up in Winnipeg. It was a decision I'd made with my high-school sweetheart, behind my parents' backs. Every few months, I would sneak off to a community health clinic near my dance studio and pick up my supply of birth control before heading into class. I popped those little white pills day in and day out. I figured someday, when I was ready, I would go off the pill and make babies. No one ever told me it might not be so straightforward.

Life on hormones was all I had ever known. My body, at least in its adult years, had never done its thing. It never ran as nature designed. I was so busy trying to avoid getting pregnant that I didn't properly understand how to get pregnant. I hadn't ever considered the consistency of my cervical fluid. I had never taken stock of how it gets slippery, like egg whites, when I ovulate, to help the sperm make its way to the egg. I hadn't ever thought about how long sperm or eggs can survive before fertilization, about how a fertilized egg makes its way through a fallopian tube, about how it embeds in the uterine lining, about the hormones that make all this possible.

When Dan and I got married in the summer of 2015, I was thirty-one and ready to go off the pill and start trying for a baby. But Dan wasn't in a rush. He wanted to wait a year or so before trying to conceive. It felt so clichéd. The woman wanting a baby sooner than the man. In the summer of 2016, when we were both ready, I went off the pill. I started having regular cycles within a few months.

Around this time, I got a debilitating concussion that, among a host of other symptoms, left me unfathomably sensitive to light and sound. Hearing a fork touch a plate caused me internal chaos. The ticking of a clock made me want to rip it off the wall. Car headlights pierced my eyes, singed my brain. I couldn't work. I couldn't be around people other than Dan. I couldn't be out in the real world. I hibernated in the quiet dimness of our home. I became incredibly anxious that anything I did would trigger new or worse symptoms. I was terrified that I might never feel whole again. I started taking an antidepressant to tamp down my anxious and dark thoughts, making sure it was considered safe for pregnancy and breastfeeding should I still need the meds by the time we conceived.

I didn't fully appreciate until around this time the extent to which I had gone through my life with some level of baseline anxiety, or generalized anxiety, as my therapist put it. It was never paralyzing. I never had any kind of breakdown or acute mental-health event. It was more of a chipping-away kind of anxiety. The ruminating kind. Not so much "The sky is falling," but "Should I?" or "What if?" It should have come as no surprise, then, that my anxiety had ramped up as I recovered from the concussion.

It can take about four to six weeks for an antidepressant to kick in, but within days I felt a sense of relief. I'm sure it was a placebo effect. I was no longer alone in the duel with my mind; the medication was there now, too, gearing up to short-circuit the thought loops I had spent years drilling into my brain.

Dan and I weren't trying to get pregnant at this point, but we weren't not trying. I wasn't tracking my cycle to make sure we were having sex during my fertile window—the roughly six-day window around the time of ovulation, during which sperm and eggs can find each other. But we were intimate often enough that we were likely to have sex at the right time. One Friday in early January of 2017, my breasts a bit sore and my period a day late, I took a pregnancy test. Our hearts beating, we watched as the hourglass on the digital test blinked until the words popped up and stared us in the face: Pregnant 1–2 Weeks. *Holy shit. I'm pregnant. We're going to have a baby.*

It was the moment that so many people dream of, that I had dreamed of. The start of a precious secret that's yours to keep and yours to share. We wanted to hold it tight, feeling intuitively protective despite our ignorance of the chances that it could go sideways. By this point, some of our closest friends were pregnant or had welcomed their first baby. I had watched their bellies swell with new life, wondering what it would feel like to grow a body inside my own. I had been to baby showers and children's birthdays, taking in the celebrations with a sense of anticipation—at some point soon it would be our turn. I had fantasized about a tiny voice calling me Mama, about being needed by someone in such a profound and consuming way.

My doctor confirmed the pregnancy by checking the level of human chorionic gonadotropin (hCG) in my blood. The hormone is created by tissue found in embryos and, in time, is produced by the placenta. While the range of potentially good hCG levels at various stages of pregnancy is quite broad, and while the rate of its increase varies from person to person and pregnancy to pregnancy, the hCG level in a healthy early pregnancy will definitely rise from one test to the next. Conventional wisdom is that it will roughly double every two days or so for much of the first trimester. Our first round of bloodwork looked good.

They say a woman becomes a mother the minute she finds out she's pregnant. In the days following the positive test, I would close my eyes, put my hand on my stomach and feel an innate connection to the cluster of cells living in my body. I knew it wasn't yet a baby, and I knew it knew nothing of me. It wasn't any bigger than a poppyseed. But my goodness did I love that poppyseed. It felt like a close and natural companion. A part of me but also distinct. I could already picture our baby, our life, our entire future. I couldn't put a face to it. It wasn't that literal. It was more of a feeling that my body was no longer mine alone.

It was also a mindfuck. Early pregnancy tends to have that effect. Either you're tired and nauseous and wishing you weren't, or you're not tired and you're not nauseous and you're wishing you were because then you'd be somewhat reassured that all was well. Other than my breasts feeling a little more tender than usual, I didn't feel particularly pregnant. I was maybe a bit tired, but I wasn't nauseous.

After a walk on a nature trail near our house one day, I flipped through my copy of *Expecting Better: Why the Conventional Pregnancy Wisdom Is Wrong—and What You Really Need to Know*, written by Brown University economist Emily Oster. It's a must-read for those trying to conceive and for those who are pregnant for the first time. It debunks myths (thou shalt not have any caffeine or wine while pregnant; sushi is bad; you can tell if it's a boy or a girl based on the fetal heartbeat), and it provides data-driven analysis on key topics such as prenatal testing, exercise, miscarriage, medications during pregnancy, diet, and pain management during labour. I skipped to the section on nausea, eager to see what Oster had to say. "As unpleasant as it is, nausea is a sign of a healthy pregnancy," she wrote. "Miscarriage rates are much lower for women who are nauseated than for those who are not." I clung to this bit: "The average pregnant woman starts to feel bad at around six weeks (that's two weeks after her missed period)." I hadn't yet hit six weeks, and I was hoping that when I did, I would feel wretched.

My doctor sent me for a second round of bloodwork to confirm that the pregnancy was progressing as it should. Before heading to the lab, I decided to pop into a nearby department store to see if they had any throw pillows for our couch. I scoped out the shelves, considering all the sizes and shapes and fabrics. As I reached for a beige pillow, an intense cramp came over me. I braced a shelf for support, nearly buckled by the sudden pain. When the wave of cramping subsided, I found the nearest washroom and locked myself in a stall, hands trembling.

I pulled down my jeans and looked at my underwear. No blood. I took that as a good sign. After I peed, though, the bright red blood started coming. "No, no, no, no," I whispered. "Please no. Please." Although bleeding in early pregnancy is relatively common—about a quarter of women will bleed in the first trimester—most miscarriages start this way. I could feel the tears welling in my eyes, waiting for me to let them spill out. I left the stall and called Dan, my voice quivering as I told him what was happening. He was concerned but also said we needed to speak with my doctor. Maybe everything was fine.

The unfortunate reality was that everything was not fine. Bloodwork confirmed I was miscarrying. "You didn't do anything wrong, honey," my doctor told me when we went in to see her for the results and talk about what would happen next. She looked me square in the eye. She knew I needed to hear her words. I clutched a tissue, wet with snot and tears and the sweat of my clammy hands. Dan had his arm around me, his knee bouncing as it does when he's nervous or uncomfortable. "Sometimes this happens, and we don't know why," she said. In her experience with patients, one in three or four pregnancies ends in a miscarriage. "Go home, eat some comfort food and crawl into bed," she said. I would likely be able to manage the bleeding and cramping from home with Tylenol and a heating pad.

I remember leaving the doctor's office and standing on the sidewalk with Dan. I leaned on the post of a stop sign, eyes downcast, shoulders slumped. I blamed myself. It was something I did. Something I ate. Something I thought. The ability of a woman to convince herself that she somehow caused a miscarriage is a thing of marvel. I would never indulge a friend thinking this way, and yet here I was allowing this to go on in my own mind. It doesn't help that even the word *miscarriage* implies the person carrying the pregnancy did something wrong. *Mis*carried, *lost* the pregnancy. I made a *mis*take and *lost* the baby. It was on *me* that the pregnancy ended. It was *my* body that shut it down, that expelled it with such bloody drama. I was so sad, so angry, so confused. So mean to myself.

I knew from Oster's book that the vast majority of miscarriages in the first trimester are a result of chromosome problems. Of the thousands of eggs that could have been released during ovulation, maybe I just so happened to have ovulated a "bad" one. I knew it was probably terrible luck. But why me? Why did I have to be one of the women who miscarries? Why hadn't we started trying to conceive sooner? Sitting on our staircase after the appointment, head in my hands sobbing, I said something along those lines to Dan. I was trying to confer on him some of the culpability I had doused so liberally on myself. It was a cruel and hurtful thing to say. This was nobody's fault and I knew that, but I didn't *know* that.

None of my close friends had experienced a miscarriage. They had gotten pregnant quickly and had their fairytale, uncomplicated pregnancies. They might not describe them as fairytale—they were nauseous, they had back pain, they were exhausted, their skin broke out, they couldn't sleep—but they had been uncomplicated nonetheless. I felt unlucky. I felt alone. I wondered if there was something very wrong with me, something that would doom every pregnancy henceforth. There was no reason to believe this was the case, but I wasn't thinking rationally.

After a few days, the cramping and bleeding stopped. My breasts were no longer tender. It was over, physically. I had passed the miscarriage naturally. No need for medical or surgical intervention. "I was so happy," I remember saying to Dan. "I'm lucky I got the chance to be pregnant, even if it was so brief, because what if that never happens again? It was the best feeling. I was so happy." Losing the pregnancy confirmed for me just how badly I wanted to become a mother, how blissful pregnancy could be. I told myself the pregnancy wasn't meant to be, that it wasn't our time. It wasn't our baby. It's common to do this, to tell ourselves stories to make ourselves feel better, to give purpose to our loss or to at least explain it.

As part of my effort to stay present and positive during my concussion recovery, I had been keeping a journal. One of the daily prompts was to list three things I was grateful for. In the days after finding out we were pregnant, I wrote things like "the news on Friday" and "the anticipation/possibility" and "the hope I feel." What was I grateful for now? "My husband's support and love, our ability to conceive, my parents' and sister's compassion," I wrote. They were the only people I could bring myself to tell right away. My parents had just happened to have flown in from British Columbia to visit my brother and me in Toronto. They had barely taken off their shoes in our entryway before I threw my arms around them, sobbing, and told them of our loss. I was broken. The concussion and miscarriage had sucked the life out of me. It was hard for them to see.

They themselves had never been through a miscarriage, and I was their first child to go through it. They didn't know what to say to make me feel better, but truth be told, nothing anybody said in that moment could have made me feel better. Well-intentioned people will say things like "At least you know you can conceive" or "At least it happened early in pregnancy. Imagine if it had happened later." Intellectually, those things are true. Intellectually, those words should bring comfort. And for a flash, maybe they do. But sometimes when you've had a dream ripped from your hands, you just want a minute to wallow. You want to take a beat to be as sad as you want to be, as sad as you feel in your bones. All I really wanted in the wake of a miscarriage was quiet compassion, a hug, a hand to hold.

I didn't want anyone's optimism until I was ready to be optimistic myself. I needed to somehow get there. I needed a new daily affirmation. I picked up my pen and wrote in my journal: "I am healthy and happy and capable of carrying a child that we will love deeply."

Something from Nothing

GETTING PREGNANT AFTER a miscarriage is treacherous ground. That magical pee-on-a-stick moment no longer feels so singularly transformative. It feels tentative, precarious, fleeting. Losing our first pregnancy robbed me of the experience of revelling in any pregnancy thereafter. It dulled the joy. It amplified the anxiety. It changed it entirely.

So, when we found out I was pregnant again in May 2017, we allowed ourselves only to be cautiously optimistic. I was hesitant to do as my friends had done and download an app to track the pregnancy week by week from the get-go. It would tell me how far along I was, roughly how big the fetus should be measuring, what changes in my body I could expect that upcoming week, and what exactly was happening in terms of the baby's development. I let myself do so only after the first ultrasound, at around seven weeks, which confirmed there was a heartbeat and that the growth was on track. This was my second pregnancy but the first time we had seen a flickering heartbeat. I held our sonogram to my chest, closed my eyes and prayed this time would be different. I let myself start to feel attached to the pregnancy, understanding that once a heartbeat was detected, the chance of miscarriage drops significantly.

As the weeks went by, the cluster of cells grew from the size of a blueberry, the app told me, to the size of a raspberry, a strawberry, a lime, a plum. By the time Baby Baum was a lemon, I was out of the first trimester and the nausea was subsiding. My feet and fingers were swollen, my face was a mess of rosacea, my legs were a tangled web of bulging purple veins. And somehow I had never felt more beautiful. Life was the best it had ever been. I was in love. I was doing a job I adored. I was pregnant with our first child, a baby girl.

Our precious Sidney arrived January 17, 2018, at 18:18—an auspicious birthdate and time for us as Jews. The number eighteen represents life. We named her for Dan's grandfather, who had just weeks before passed away at the age of 101. One life had ended. Another was beginning.

I had no idea then just what a miracle she was. What a miracle we all are.

In the early fall of 2018, when Sid was about eight months old, I saw a pair of brothers playing at a park in the warmth of the sun. I know this because I wrote about it in the journal I sporadically kept at the time. The older boy was blowing bubbles and the younger one was chasing the iridescent orbs as they tumbled in the breeze and fell, trying to pop them before they hit a blade of grass or floated off into the distance. "It was so cute to see," I wrote in a September 26th entry I addressed to Sid. My mom had written letters to me when I was young, and I loved reading them as I got older. I wanted Sid to have that same experience one day, so I jotted down my thoughts sporadically. "It makes us want to give you a lil sibling ASAP. It's clichéd to say I don't care whether it's a boy or a girl, but it's true. We just want a healthy baby. A sister would be lovely, as I so cherish my relationship with your Auntie Mackenzie [my younger sister], but a boy would be fun in its own new and different way."

The idea that I ever gave thought to whether Sid's sibling would be a boy or a girl, as if that mattered one bit, as if I had any control, would be laughable if it wasn't so naive. Even after the experience of a miscarriage before Sid was conceived, I was unaware of all the ways another viable pregnancy might not happen for us. About a week later, I wrote her another note: "I'm supposed to get my period today, at the latest. I really hope I'm pregnant. Would love to give you a little brother or sister so close in age. Chances are I'm not pregnant . . . but a girl can hope." I took a pregnancy test a couple of days later. Only one line appeared. Not pregnant.

To say I was hung up on having children close in age would be a massive understatement. I became borderline obsessive. Which is so bizarre because I'm one of five children in a tight-knit blended family where the age difference between the youngest and the eldest is fully twelve years. I'm six years older than my only sister, Mackenzie. Despite this age gap, she's my closest friend, my person. We talk every day. I'm also very close with my three brothers: One is nine years younger than me, one is two months older than me, and the other is three years older than me. I know from personal experience that siblings don't need to be close in age to be close. So why was I so obsessed with firing out babies so quickly?

I've scrutinized this idea since going through fertility treatment. I'm not sure I thought much about it beforehand or in the midst. Did I *actually* care if my kids were close in age? Did *I* really truly care? Or was I simply going along to the beat of society's drum, which has conditioned us to plot our lives such that we're pregnant with our second child not long after we celebrate our first's first birthday? Was this some kind of manifestation of my competitive spirit? Of wanting to keep up with my friends? With strangers even? "Two under two," people would post on social media. I wanted two under two, but I'm not convinced that was a conscious or original thought.

I can't even say with clarity when it was that I knew I wanted to be a mother, for that matter. I suppose it was always the case. I took for granted that I wanted to have children, and it just so happened that I truly did. I never interrogated why the feeling was there; I just knew I felt it. I wonder now about the degree to which my yearning to become a mother was rooted in my upbringing, in my experience being a child myself. My childhood wasn't perfect, but it was full of love and laughter and closeness. Perhaps there was something in me that wanted to recreate that feeling of a unit, to be the foundation for a family the way my parents were. When it came to wanting a second child, I think it was some combination of primal desire, personal experience with my own siblings, social pressure and personality that drove both Dan and me to forge ahead.

Unfortunately or fortunately, we're stubborn people. Dan is the kind of person who won't stop until he finishes what he started. He has trouble putting down a book if he's partway through a chapter. He. Must. Finish. The. Chapter. He's a Taurus, the sign of the bull. My school report cards, beginning at an early age, consistently featured the word *determined*. I had always felt that if I worked hard enough, I could achieve what I set out to accomplish. "When you're trying to have a baby, you're at the mercy of forces outside your control," Dan reflected years later. "It's incredibly humbling."

Of course, it makes sense to have children close in age if it's a matter of the woman's age and fertility. It's also perhaps easier to do things as a family if the kids are at similar stages, at least at the beginning. It might be nice to move on from the bottles, strollers and cribs. The relationship in the kids' younger years may be more tightly bonded. But these are fleeting and subjective advantages. To want a small age gap for the sake of having a small age gap is not reason enough alone. And yet when we deviate from the timeline of having children more or less back to back, we're liable to feel separate and apart from the masses, especially when that includes our inner circle of loved ones who occupy the most space in our brains, hearts and calendars.

Even if I had no intrinsic reason to want kids close in age, I can say for certain that I had a deep desire to give Sid a sibling. Those brothers in the park that September day stirred up memories from a childhood spent laughing, playing, chasing and being chased.

Born and raised in Winnipeg, Manitoba, with my brothers and sister, I always had someone to talk to, play with, fight with, compete with, conspire with, laugh with, confide in. People were constantly coming and going from our house. There was always a critical mass to keep our home at a base level of lively. We didn't need to make plans with friends to fill our evenings or weekends because our house was already full. We didn't need to bring friends on our family ski trips because we had each other. Looking back now on those road trips across the Prairies to the Rockies, I wonder how my parents stayed sane. (It's likely they didn't.) Three boys and two girls packed into a van and an SUV, ski gear practically spilling out the roof rack, pillows and blankets strewn on the crumb-filled rows of seats, Yahtzee dice rolling around on the floor.

When people asked how many kids Dan and I had, we used to say "just Sid" or "just one." Maybe I was being overly sensitive, but it felt as if people didn't expect us to have "only one" kid. Because that would mean our family wasn't "complete." It wouldn't be the way it "should" be. At some point along the way, I realized the framing of "just one" didn't feel good. I started saying "We have one" or "It's the three of us." Most people knew better than to prod. Others would explicitly ask if we were trying for another. (If you're one of those people, stop being that person.) We had our response in the can—some version of "Right now, it's the three of us," "We'll see," "Who knows."

As time went on, that canned response became the truth. Who knew?

I'm speaking softly in the video. Sidney is asleep down the hall, and Dan and I are lying in bed, eyes still heavy in the morning light. Arm extended over us, I've got my phone camera turned on us as we say the news out loud, wanting to capture the moment. "We just found out that I'm pregnant," I said with a smile, holding up a pregnancy test to the camera. "I'm whispering because our other little baby is sleeping. It's March 17, Sidney's fourteen-month birthday." We were thrilled. We had just started properly trying for a second child and were relieved we had conceived so quickly. We kept the news to ourselves, wanting to get through the first trimester or at least further into it. An experience with a miscarriage does that to you. It brings alive the statistics and makes them personal.

We kept busy. I took Sid to watch her dad play hockey in an intramural league. We visited with my older brother and his family. We had my younger brother and his wife over to spend time with Sid. We tried to teach her how to walk. We threw Dan's mom a seventy-fifth birthday party. We went to a farmers' market with friends. We took Sid to the park, where I pushed her and Dan on a giant saucer swing.

Going back through photos from this time, I see that I had some spotting on April 2 and 3, 2019. These are the kinds of pictures you have in your camera roll if you've ever had a miscarriage—bloody evidence on a panty liner to text your partner or to show to a doctor in case you're asked what, exactly, the spotting looked like. Was it brown? Was it red? Was it clotted? It was brown, which I knew was better than bright red. I reminded myself that some spotting in early pregnancy is perfectly normal.

Our first ultrasound was a few days later, on the morning of April 9. There was a heartbeat. Based on the date of the first day of my most recent period, I should have been seven weeks and six days pregnant, or 7w6d, as the ultrasound monitor showed in shorthand. I always thought that was strange. A woman is never one or two or three weeks pregnant. The count starts at four weeks. Four weeks from the start of your most recent period. If you were due to get your period on April 1 and you pee on a stick on April 29 and it's positive, you're considered four weeks pregnant. A full-term pregnancy is forty weeks—that's ten months, not nine months as we've learned. That first month literally happens before you know it.

The blob on the ultrasound was measuring a few days smaller than it should have been based on the start of my last menstrual cycle. We were asked to come back a week later to make sure it was growing as it should. The days moved slowly as we waited to go back for the follow-up ultrasound. The test showed a week's worth of growth, so we were back to being optimistic. The technician gave us a sonogram image to take home. The little babe looked like a gummy bear. We started calling it Teddy.

Around this time, one of my closest friends, who had her first daughter just two weeks after we had Sid, called me from the United States. She was pregnant too. We were both due in November, though I wasn't yet ready to reciprocate with our own news.

That weekend, we went up to the cottage with Dan's family, about a two-hour drive northeast of Toronto. We hadn't told anyone about the pregnancy. I wasn't feeling particularly nauseous or tired, so it wasn't so difficult to hide. Sid was playing with her older cousins when I went to use the washroom. I wasn't having any cramping; I wasn't particularly on edge. I was caught off guard, then, when I stood up from the toilet and saw blood in the bowl. Dark clots and strings of thick blood started slipping out of me, sinking into the water like an oil spill. I sat back down, in shock. We had *just* seen Teddy's heartbeat flickering on the ultrasound a couple of days earlier.

I called Dan upstairs and showed him the scene in the toilet. We started Googling, plugging in searches like *bleeding in early pregnancy*; *just saw heartbeat but bleeding 8w pregnant*; *bleeding but no cramping early pregnancy*; *blood clots early pregnancy*. The internet told us that perhaps the bleeding was the result of a subchorionic hematoma, a collection of blood under the membrane that attaches the uterine wall to the amniotic sac. Most subchorionic hematomas, marked as an SCH on an ultrasound report, will resolve on their own and won't cause pregnancy complications. Maybe that's what this was?

But then the cramping started. I was familiar with the feeling. We decided to get in the car and drive an hour to the hospital in Peterborough. Our family was shocked. It was hard to process the prospect of a miscarriage when they hadn't even known I was pregnant. As Dan and I wove along the country roads to the highway, we listened to folk music—the kind that could make you cry on a good day. We held hands the entire time, palms clammy with nerves, pits in our stomachs.

We checked in at the emergency room and were sent downstairs for an ultrasound. Dan waited outside the room while I climbed onto the exam table, the white paper crinkling beneath me as I slid my body into place. I explained why we were there as the technician prepped the probe with ultrasound gel and then inserted it. "Is there a heartbeat?" I asked, panicked. She told me she needed to do her assessment and that the doctor would talk to us afterward. I looked up at the ceiling, tears in my eyes, holding my breath. I had to remind myself to breathe. I tried to read her face, but she wouldn't look at me. When she did, it was over, her expression showing what I read as pity. I hoped I was wrong.

When we were called in to go over the results, I couldn't focus on what the doctor was saying because I could see the paperwork in his hands. Handwritten in black pen were the words *spontaneous abortion.* I burst into tears. "It wasn't like it was a baby," the doctor said. "You were only about eight or nine weeks. It's not much of anything at that point." Not much of anything? Not much of anything? It was something to us. It was already *someone* to us. I was so angry at him I could have screamed.

Dan took my arm, and we made our way out of the hospital. The moment the fresh air and sunlight hit my face, my legs buckled beneath me. I dropped to the cold damp cement, head between my knees as I lost my breath to the heartbreak. "I can't," I cried, Dan wrapping his arms around me. "I can't do this again." But what choice did we have? The world doesn't stop when you miscarry. A life ended inside you, but life must go on. We got into the car and made our way back to the cottage, my vision blurry with tears. Dan wouldn't let go of my hand, squeezing it to reassure me that we would get through this together. That we could run through walls together. His mom, sisters and nieces were waiting at the door when we arrived, looking at us with the same pity I had seen in the technician's eyes. Sid was on her aunt's hip.

I said nothing, my gaze downcast. I had to keep it together. I scooped Sid into my arms and held her tight, breathing her in. She was my life raft. I was holding on to one baby for dear life while I let another go.

Miscarriages are fickle things. Everyone's experience is different, so no one can really tell you what to expect, beyond warning of some cramping and bleeding. But how bad will that cramping be? Will it be crippling? Will you need to go to the hospital? Most women manage a miscarriage at home, using pads to soak up the blood and a hot compress to soothe the tummy. But the truth is who knows. The level of pain or blood loss isn't always correlated to gestational age. You can have a gory, horribly painful miscarriage at six weeks. You can have what's called a missed miscarriage at twelve weeks, in which you experience no physical signs that the pregnancy has spontaneously shut down.

And why do they happen in the first place? Genetic issues with the embryo account for about two-thirds of early losses. "The majority of losses happen because of random genetic bad luck," Dr. Sony Sierra, a reproductive endocrinologist who co-runs the recurrent pregnancy loss program at Toronto's Trio Fertility, told me. "As you get older, it's more common, but even young people will have losses because of random bad luck. When you have more than two losses, the chances it was random bad luck decreases and the chance that it's something else is higher. After two losses, it's appropriate to start to investigate other causes . . . especially if there are any other gynecologic issues going on or if you're older than thirty-five." Those two losses, she explained, don't need to be consecutive. At the time, we had no idea we had officially entered complicated ground.

My second miscarriage was more painful and bloodier than my first. A few days after I started passing the pregnancy, I was slated to leave with Sid for Kelowna, British Columbia, where my parents, sister and one of my brothers live. My mom and I were throwing my sister a baby shower to celebrate the recent birth of her first child, a boy. I knew it would be hard to go on my own (Dan had a work trip scheduled for the same time), but I wanted to be there. I was of the mind that just because something bad happens doesn't mean we don't celebrate the good.

I got off the plane in Kelowna and handed Sid to my dad the moment I saw him waiting for us in the baggage area. My black leggings were soaked through with blood. I got clean underwear and pants out of my suitcase and changed my pad. The blood was still coming in fits and starts. Just when I thought that was the last of it, more would come. When I emerged from the bathroom, my dad hugged me extra tight, held me longer than usual. He knew his girl was hurting. My dad is my hero, my rock. I needed his arms around me. I needed his comfort.

After getting settled at my parents' place, I set about helping with the decorations for the shower. The theme was the book *Guess How Much I Love You* by Sam McBratney, a classic and a family favourite. I muscled through mounting the bunny bunting, plating the glazed carrot-shaped cookies, arranging the white peonies. When the time came, I put on the dress that I had weeks before thought might show off a little bump. I should have been about ten weeks along. I should have been making small talk with Mackenzie's friends while keeping a joyful secret. Instead, I was harbouring a different kind of secret, a sad and ongoing one that was still making its way through me.

I held my nephew and tried not to cry, consumed by his soft skin and newborn smell. Research has shown that the scent of a newborn can feel as good as a hit of drugs to an addict—a rush of dopamine, the activation of the neurological reward circuit. My sister and I didn't take a single photo together that day, which is entirely unlike us. In the few photos that I am in, I look pale and drained.

It's hard to know whether my decision to go to the shower was "good" or "bad," whether it was buoying or an act of self-harm. These days, there are fertility mindset coaches who can help people move through these kinds of decisions. Emily Getz is one of them. The Toronto-based mother and former IVF patient runs Day 1 Fertility, a support network that includes coaching, community and a podcast. Getz comes to the work with her own trials and tribulations. In 2019, when her first-born son was two years old, she had a late-term pregnancy loss and delivered a stillborn baby girl, Ruby, at twenty-three weeks. She spent the next five years trying with all her might to give her son a sibling. She had been through the wringer, from an ectopic pregnancy, which caused her to lose one of her fallopian tubes, to multiple miscarriages, several egg retrievals and failed embryo transfers. She finally got viably pregnant in late 2024 using a donor egg and delivered a baby girl in May 2025.

I went for a walk with Getz in the fall of 2023, while she was still in the throes of her secondary-infertility journey. We meandered through a ravine, exchanging war stories. The way she sees it, fertility patients are carrying around an invisible backpack full of bricks, weighed down by worries and anxieties. Some of those worries and anxieties have to be in the backpack. They're just part of the deal; there's no real way of getting around it. The risk of miscarriage. The possibility of a failed embryo transfer. The hormonal toll of medications. As patients, we have to learn how to carry the backpack, to be resilient, to build the strength to bear the load. Some of those bricks, though, are movable. The weight doesn't have to be so heavy.

One such brick is the age-gap brick. We add it to our backpack ourselves, or we let others do it for us—our friends, family, societal forces. That goddamn brick causes so much pain. We usually only get over it because we have to. The passage of time forces us to. And then once we do, we feel lighter. For those trying to have their first child, there's the left-behind brick for the feeling of being left out as loved ones welcome babies.

I spoke with one woman who recalled how she found out her younger brother was expecting a baby, while she was in the midst of an arduous fertility journey. "Instead of telling me in a quiet place or in a text or phone call, they told me on Mother's Day at a restaurant with the rest of our family present," she recounted. "They gave us gifts: mugs that said Best Auntie Ever, Best Granddad Ever. I had to hold my shit together. Everyone was looking at me. I went into the bathroom, had a tiny cry, let a little out. When we got into our car, I started bawling, snot streaming down my face. I felt the frustration in all of the cells of my body."

It's true that we can be happy for someone else and upset for ourselves. We're not bad people for feeling sadness and envy at every pregnancy announcement and baby shower that's not our own. We're not horrible for having an easier time being happy for someone who finally got pregnant after a tough road than we do for someone who came to it easily. It feels shitty, but *we're* not shitty. It's human nature. It's natural to compare ourselves to others, but that doesn't mean we shouldn't do our very best to see our life right in front us. *Our* life, and no one else's. Dan was exceptional at that. He knows that comparison is the thief of joy. When I was low, I said to him that I was sorry, that if he were with someone else, maybe he wouldn't have had to endure losses, maybe he would have all his children by now. He took my cheeks in his hands. "I wouldn't trade my life with you for anything or anyone," he said. They say if we all threw our problems in a pile and saw everyone else's, we'd scramble to pick our own back up. There he was, seeing our problem in the pile and picking it back up, picking me back up.

Mackenzie would have understood if I cancelled the trip or opted to sit out the baby shower. I'm so glad I didn't, because I got to see the depths of her kindness, graciousness and sensitivity. She was careful with her words, understated with her joy. She knew how to be around me. She knew how to make me feel better without making me feel worse. That's what a sibling is for. That's why I would fight so hard.

My Roman Empire

AFTER A MISCARRIAGE, all you want is for your hCG to go back down to zero. Zero means it's over. Zero means you'll likely get a period in four to eight weeks. Zero means you can try again soon. How soon depends on a few factors, including how far along you were when you had the loss. It also depends on who you ask. There was a time when doctors recommended waiting a year before trying again. The World Health Organization still advises waiting six months. These days, though, clinicians tend to say that, in general, so long as a person has had a normal period after a loss, they can try again when they're emotionally ready to do so.

My bloodwork showed that my hCG was dropping, but then it plateaued, refusing to get to nil. There had to be some pregnancy tissues lingering in my uterus—retained products of conception, as doctors call them. I felt suffocated in my own body, claustrophobic. I wanted to get the death out of me. I knew it wasn't a dead baby in there, but it was a dead dream and I wanted it gone. I wanted it out. I felt sick at the thought of my body harbouring those cells. I was mad at it for shutting down the pregnancy. And now I was mad at it for not getting rid of it fast enough.

Unlike with my first loss, the natural route to pass the pregnancy wasn't working. This left me with two options to manage the miscarriage: medically or surgically. The medical approach typically involves taking a two-drug combination called Mifegymiso, which is comprised of mifepristone and misoprostol. Mifepristone decreases progesterone and causes uterine contractions, and misoprostol helps the cervix soften and dilate to release the tissues. The pregnancy is usually expelled within about forty-eight hours of starting the protocol. The surgical option involves aspirating the tissues through gentle suctioning or through a D&C, which is the same dilation and curettage procedure that's used in surgical abortions.

As it happened, I had in 2017 written an article for *The Globe and Mail* about Mifegymiso, colloquially known as the abortion pill. The drug had been approved in more than sixty countries, including the United States and China, by the time it landed on the Canadian market. It made headlines in the context of representing a sea change in how women in Canada could choose to end their pregnancies, but the drug combo can also be used to manage miscarriages before about nine weeks gestation.

Medication is believed to be about 85 percent successful in clearing a miscarriage. In the rest of the cases, tissues remain and surgical intervention is required. A D&C, meantime, is somewhere in the order of 97 percent effective in removing tissues from the uterus. I wanted this behind me. And I definitely didn't want to take the meds and end up needing a D&C anyhow.

My doctor referred me to the women's unit at a downtown hospital, where I would be assessed for a potential D&C. On May 14, 2019, we met with a compassionate nurse who talked us through what the procedure would entail. Doctors would put me under general anesthesia, dilate my cervix and then scrape the lining of my uterus to remove the retained tissues. The meeting is a blur to me. I'm sure she went over the risks, and I'm sure I signed a document acknowledging them. I don't remember anything about the possibility of developing scar tissue in my uterus that could prevent me from carrying another pregnancy to term, though it's entirely plausible she told us about the risk of developing postoperative uterine adhesions and I simply didn't register the gravity. What I recall vividly is coming away from the conversation feeling like a D&C was the quickest way to move on. We opted to go ahead with the procedure at the hospital.

The D&C was booked for two days later. I packed a little bag for the hospital. Socks because the nurse said the OR area is chilly. A phone charger. Loose-fitting clothes for afterward. When I arrived in the surgical area, I put my belongings in a locker and changed into a blue hospital gown. I asked for a blanket. It was cold. A nurse brought over a thick, pilling white sheet with blue stripes and draped it over me. An IV was inserted into a vein on my arm, around the crease of my elbow. It burned as it went in, a pang of pain as the nurse adjusted the line. The doctor explained what would transpire. He also noted that there had been a request to test the tissue for genetic abnormalities. This was something he personally didn't think was necessary. This was *only* my second miscarriage, and I had *only* been eight or nine weeks along. I felt guilty for requesting it, as if I had somehow inconvenienced everyone by having a miscarriage and wanting to know why it happened.

My eyes filled with tears, the lump in my throat all but choking me as I looked up at the ceiling and drifted off to sleep.

The decision to go ahead with a D&C at the hospital was, for a long time, my Roman Empire. It was the thing that frequently occupied my thoughts, lived rent-free in my mind. To me, there was BD&C and AD&C. Before the D&C and after it. Founded or not—it's impossible to know for sure—I believed for years that the procedure was detrimental. It's where I drew a line in the sand of our fertility journey.

Now, I'm not so sure. Now, I wonder if it was less about the procedure itself and more about the circumstances under which it was performed.

As with a lot of topics in fertility, the subject of D&Cs is dizzying. Should you get one after a miscarriage? How and where should it be performed? At a hospital? At a fertility clinic? There's no simple answer because it all depends on your personal situation. Thousands of D&Cs are performed each year in the United States alone, for abortion and for miscarriage management. They can be life-saving in cases involving postnatal hemorrhage. The vast majority of patients who undergo a D&C will be fine, at least physically. But for those who end up with significant scar tissue in their uterus, the procedure could mean never carrying a baby. It's hard to know how often D&Cs lead to adhesions, because it's uncommon for doctors or their patients to assess the uterus for scar tissue after the procedure.

For years, I questioned whether I should have gotten a D&C. Whether I should have pushed to have it done using ultrasound guidance and gentle suctioning at a fertility clinic where my reproductive future would be top of mind. For years, I was angry with myself for not asking more questions.

I'm not alone in my obsession with my D&C as a turning point. I spoke with several women who said they went ahead with the procedure because they were desperate to move forward and start trying again.

One woman I spoke with said she was advised to take misoprostol—never told of the Mifegymiso combo—after a loss at around seven weeks. An ultrasound later showed that the medication hadn't been entirely successful; there were retained products from the naturally conceived pregnancy. "I was told I should have a D&C," she said. "I wasn't really told of the risks. I think of this day and I wince at myself."

Before the procedure at a women's clinic, she spoke with an on-site counsellor who reassured her that she was doing the right thing, that she would be a mother someday. After the D&C, she was sent on her way, told she would get a period again in the next month or so, that starting her menstrual cycle would be her indication that this saga was behind her, that she could start trying again. Except that her period didn't come. Except that she ended up needing a surrogate to carry her child. The scarring was too significant.

"I would encourage women to slow down," she told me.

"Yesterday went as well as could be expected," I emailed the nurse the day after the D&C. "More than anything, I feel relieved." I wanted her to know how much I appreciated her humanity. "A friend of mine saw you a couple of years ago after a miscarriage and was singing your praises. As was I!" I wrote. "You really truly are doing what you're meant to do. Thank you for being so kind and patient with us women when we're at such a fragile point in life. Let me know what's next, so we can get on to baby-making again."

Fragile.

I often felt like an inconvenience, particularly in the health-care system. Sorry to cry. Sorry to ask. Sorry to bug you. Sorry, but. I was self-conscious about my pain, emotional and physical. I didn't want to complain too much about any of it. Many people had been through this, were going through this, would go through this. I wasn't special. The hormones were coursing through me, but God forbid I come across as hormonal. God forbid I embody the trope of the hysterical woman who can't control her emotions. For centuries, hysteria was considered a female disorder. The word, in fact, comes from the Greek word for uterus. In a hysterical woman, a barren, untethered uterus roams through her body, wreaking all kinds of havoc. Anxiety, insomnia, depression, irritability and fainting spells.

A woman was considered predisposed to being crazy by sheer virtue of having a uterus and, worse yet, an empty one.

It was hard to shake the voices of the doctor who informed me of my miscarriage and the doctor who did my D&C. Their words diminished my experience and my emotions around it. *I shouldn't have been that sad. I shouldn't want more information. It was just a minor procedure. Nothing to see here.* Honestly, fuck them and fuck that. These two doctors, both men, had absolutely no business judging my reaction to losing a pregnancy. The way they handled me in those vulnerable moments set the tone for how I thought I should behave as a woman going through a fertility journey. I wish I could face them now, tell them that the miscarriage and the subsequent "minor" procedure set off a chain of events that nearly robbed us of the chance at another child. How's that for dramatic, hysterical?

In early June, the nurse sent us the genetic testing report of the retained tissues removed during the D&C. It stated that the result for the specimen was "abnormal" and "consistent with triploidy in a male." Male. A boy. What could have been a brother for Sid. The nurse pointed us to an entry on the National Organization for Rare Disorders website, to help us better understand the finding. We clicked on it right away.

> Triploidy is a rare chromosomal abnormality. Triploidy is the presence of an additional set of chromosomes in the cell for a total of 69 chromosomes rather than the normal 46 chromosomes per cell. The extra set of chromosomes originates either from the father or the mother during fertilization. Pregnancies with triploidy are usually miscarried early in the pregnancy. If the pregnancy continues to term, the infant dies within the first days of life. . . . A few affected individuals have been reported to have survived to adulthood,

but had developmental delay, learning difficulties, seizures, hearing loss and other abnormalities.

It sounded horrible. It also made me feel a thousand times better. There was nothing I did or didn't do that caused the miscarriage. My body had done the right thing. That feeling lasted a few seconds. Because then I read the rest of the report, which said the test indicated that the extra set of chromosomes came from me.

A couple of days later, the nurse let me know that my hCG was finally less than one. I was considered back to baseline. "Yay!" I emailed Dan from the newsroom. "Only news that would have been better is that I was pregnant lol." He responded a few minutes later: "Haha one step at a time:)"

With my hCG down to zero, we were back to trying. I used a digital fertility monitor to help us pinpoint when I was ovulating, peeing on the test sticks every morning. If the monitor showed Peak on the screen, it was time to have sex. We became laser-focused on getting pregnant again. I thought of my days in terms of the menstrual phases, because it helped make every day of the month feel productive. There was Having My Period, there was Eggs Growing, there was Ovulating, there was the Two-Week Wait until a pregnancy might be detected.

Going through my emails from around this time, I see myself becoming more and more anxious and more and more fixated on having a baby. Over the course of two weeks in August, I wrote the nurse at the hospital multiple times. To find out if it was safe to use a topical medication to treat a stye in my eye. (We were in the Two-Week Wait.) To ask why, even though I was two days late for my period, the pregnancy tests kept coming back negative. Occam's razor: The simplest explanation is usually the correct one. I wasn't pregnant.

My Google searches in those days were rife with questions, most of them pretty reaching, pretty in the weeds. How long does an egg last? How soon after fertilization might I feel something? How long can sperm survive inside me? How soon could I test to see if I was pregnant? How do I know if the spotting I'm getting is the start of my period or implantation bleeding, caused by the embryo burrowing into my uterine lining? If I'm not getting egg-white cervical mucous, does that mean I didn't ovulate this month? Can you ovulate and not have egg whites? If I tested too early and it came back negative, what are the chances a second line will appear when I test again in twenty-four hours? Maybe I should check the test again, pull it out of the garbage and make sure it really does only have one line. Are the results still reliable? Do I have to test with my first morning urine? How early in the morning can I pee on a stick? Is there such a thing as too early?

Most of my girlfriends who were trying to conceive did no such Googling. They spoke about getting (and staying) pregnant as if it were a foregone conclusion. They made it sound so simple and straightforward, as if they could place an order for a viable pregnancy and the fertility gods would deliver.

On the evening of October 4, I looked in the mirror and noticed my skin was flaring up. Pink rosacea bumps had popped up around my nose and mouth. That seemed to happen whenever I got pregnant. I hadn't thought for a second I was pregnant that month, because I'd had what I thought was my period, granted a bit earlier than expected and a bit lighter than usual. My skin, though, was telling me something. Dan was out for an after-dinner walk with Sid when I decided to take a test. I had one on hand, as one does when trying to conceive.

I peed on the stick, and to my surprise, it was positive. I put on my shoes and found Dan and Sid, just down the block. I distracted him and handed Sid the test to give to him. "Dada," she said. He took the blue and white stick, looked at it, and then looked at me, perplexed, beaming. I laughed and hugged him, explaining that the light bleeding I'd had over the past few days must have been from the embryo implanting. About a quarter of pregnant women experience implantation bleeding.

I emailed the nurse right away. She had told me to do so the minute I got a positive test. The women's unit at the hospital would help me manage the early stages of the pregnancy. My hCG confirmed a pregnancy, at 391 IU/L. That initial figure in and of itself doesn't tell you much in early pregnancy. The absolute value matters, but it matters less than the rate at which it increases, particularly because it's usually hard to know the precise date of conception. My lab reports from the following day show that my hCG had gone up to 537 IU/L. The level was supposed to double every forty-eight hours or so, and it had only been one day, so that number was fine. On the lower end, but fine.

At any rate, I was pregnant. So, too, were several of the friends who had spoken so nonchalantly about their plans to make another baby. They were a couple months ahead of me, but we were all on the same track. In the days after learning we had conceived, Dan and I left for California for a friend's wedding. Our first stop when we landed in Los Angeles was In-N-Out Burger. I skipped the mayo because of the raw egg yolks. I didn't want to eat, do, think or say anything that could jeopardize the pregnancy or give me ammunition for self-blame if I miscarried. We drove along the scenic Pacific Coast Highway, windows open, feeling the warm breeze and smelling the salt of the ocean, toward Big Sur. We went for dinner, and I relished in my inability to have a drink.

We hiked Tanbark Trail in Julia Pfeiffer Burns State Park the next morning, weaving through the redwoods until we reached a waterfall. The redwood forests of California have always been special to me. The sweet, earthy smell transported me to summer hikes with my mom on dusty trails. There's something about those trees that brings me calm—their scent, their sturdy trunks, their towering stature that makes me feel small. There were swaths of the forest that had been damaged by wildfires over the years, though redwood trees stand up to blazes better than most other species. Forest fires aren't always bad. They release nutrients stored on the forest floor and promote new growth. It's Mother Nature at work. The cycle of life. The fires might leave scars, but they also usher rebirth.

After a couple nights in Big Sur, we made our way along the coast to Carmel-by-the-Sea for the wedding. I was secretly pregnant, sipping virgin vodka sodas with a wedge of lime. The morning of the wedding, I went down to the hotel pool to lie in the shade and go for a dip.

I saw a woman swimming laps and had a flashback to my time competitive swimming as a kid. I had loved it. Freestyle, breaststroke, butterfly, backstroke. All of it. I was a fish in a former life, but for some reason I hadn't gotten back into training in my adult years. I started chatting with the woman about swimming, about how meditative it is, about how life is drowned out when your head is underwater. The world sounds different. You're weightless. She offered to let me use her goggles so I could swim a few laps.

I was immediately transported. I was back at Winnipeg's Pan Am Pool, doing drills with the Manta Swim Club, feeling my hands slice through the water with each pull. One, two, three, breath, one, two, three, breath. Feet lax and fluttering just beneath the surface. I watched the rays of light cut through the water and dance on the tiles below. I had forgotten how beautiful and mesmerizing that is. I hadn't done a flip turn off the wall in I-don't-know-how-long, but muscle memory brought it back to me and there I was, training again.

Some of my earliest memories are at the pool. When I was about eight or nine years old, I wanted to swim in the deep end at a community pool. I was told I was too young to take the swim test to do so. I convinced the lifeguard on duty to let me do the test anyway. I swam the required laps no problem. The hardest part was diving to the bottom of the pool and retrieving a brick. I don't remember how deep it was, but it was deeper than I had ever dove. I propelled myself downward, the pressure building in my head as I kicked and pulled toward the bottom. When I emerged, I hoisted the brick in the air, out of breath, proud.

I thanked the woman at the hotel pool for the use of her goggles. What a treat, I told her. It was enough to pique my interest in finding a place to train in Toronto. I went up to our room to get ready for the festivities, feeling energized by my swim but also fatigued. I hoped that was a good sign.

We made our way to the ceremony on the hotel grounds. Dan squeezed my hand and I squeezed it back, our signal that he had me and I had him. We spent the evening reconnecting with friends who, after Dan's time at business school in Boston, had scattered across Canada and the United States. Part of me was there, present. But a bigger part of me was in the future, thinking of what was to come and all the what ifs. Of the due date in late spring. Of how Sid would be a bit less than two and a half years old when the baby came. Of whether it would be a boy or another girl. I also thought of losing the pregnancy. Every time I went to the bathroom, I would hold my breath, fearful that I would see blood in my underwear, on the toilet paper, in the water. I hadn't had any cramping, but I hadn't had any cramping the last time I miscarried so the absence of pain wasn't particularly reassuring.

We got back to Toronto on the Sunday of the Thanksgiving long weekend, so I waited until the Tuesday morning to go for more bloodwork to see how the hCG was tracking. I dropped off Sid at daycare, went to the lab and then headed to the newsroom and got to work. I was prepping to help cover the upcoming federal election when my phone rang. It was the nurse with my results. I left my desk and found an empty office to take the call. I shut the big glass sliding door. "I'm sorry to tell you this, but your hCG went down," she said. "What?" I said, slowly lowering myself onto a chair. "What do you mean it went down? I haven't had any cramping. No bleeding. Are you sure? This doesn't make any sense."

She was sure. My hCG had gone down to 376 IU/L. Not that the number really mattered. Down was bad. Conclusive. There was no ambiguity. We were having another loss. The news punched me in the gut and slapped me in the face. So many thoughts were racing through my mind. How could this be happening again? Why was this happening again? Did I swim too many laps? I shouldn't have done those somersaulting flip turns. I must have done something wrong. What was wrong with me? How am I going to get over this again? Can I? I don't want to break this to Dan.

The nurse tried to comfort me, but I needed to get off the phone. I was in a fishbowl office in the newsroom and wanted to escape. I could barely breathe. I felt so betrayed by my body. I needed to leave and call Dan. I snuck out of the newsroom but in my haste forgot my car key on my desk. From the lobby, I emailed a colleague to say what had happened and asked him to bring it down to me. He gave me a knowing hug. He and his husband were going through their own fertility hell. "I'm so sorry," he said.

I got into my car, shut the door and grabbed the steering wheel with both hands. I wanted something to brace against when I let out a scream.

Mother of All Invention

TO THINK, MOST people have sex to make a baby. To think, *we* had sex to make a baby. It seems so simple. So presumed. So natural. The idea that it could be literally orgasmic is unfathomable to those who have slogged through the trenches of fertility treatment, just for the chance. It should be unfathomable to us all.

Whether it was sex or modern science that put you on this earth, an absurd number of things had to go just right. From a young age, we have been taught some version of the following: Sperm meets egg, creates embryo, turns into baby, is born. That is both true and far from the whole truth. It's unnecessary here to describe in detail how it is exactly that humans reproduce. But I think it's important to at the very least have a common understanding of what it means to conceive, so we can appreciate why it doesn't always happen when and how we want it to—and so we can marvel together at its awesomeness when it does.

The established thinking is that a female developed all the eggs she will ever have as a fetus. What does this mean, practically speaking? It means the eggs that made my children were created inside their grandmother's womb. A female fetus has somewhere in the order of six million eggs. By the time she's born, that number will have fallen to a million or so. Only a few hundred thousand will survive to puberty, the rest having disintegrated within the fluid-filled follicles that host them. Natural selection at its most nascent.

At a precise time of the month, the brain releases a luteinizing hormone that travels by blood to the ovaries, telling the follicles to prepare an egg for maturation and release. While a few dozen eggs hear the call of duty and snap to action, only one emerges dominant. Only one will ovulate. The others stop growing and peter out into nothingness.

Like some kind of sci-fi creature, the empty egg follicle morphs into another entity altogether, secreting the estrogen and progesterone necessary to prepare for the potential implantation of an embryo. The uterine lining thickens in anticipation of a zygote searching for a cozy place to burrow. Finger-like tentacles at the end of a fallopian tube sweep the egg along, down toward the uterus. If the Chosen Egg isn't fertilized by sperm within about twelve to twenty-four hours, it dies, and the uterine lining is then shed as a period.

The male contribution to conception is prolific, if inefficient. Hundreds of millions of sperm are released with each ejaculation of semen—a fluid with a very specific pH level that's compatible with the acidity of a female's slick cervical mucous secreted around the time she ovulates. Only a few hundred ejaculated sperm reach the egg, helped along by a tail that propels them and by the estrogen-fuelled uterine contractions that guide them toward the Chosen Egg.

The sperm bind to the egg, their heads releasing enzymes that digest the outer shell. The Chosen Sperm—one out of the hundreds of millions from that single ejaculation—permeates the egg. The cell membranes fuse. Two become one. The fusion gives rise to a protective barrier that prevents other sperm from also fertilizing the Chosen Egg. The ultimate cock block.

The single cell, with its genetic material from the sperm and the egg, divides over and over and over and over (and over and over to the power of over and over) to form a raspberry-like cluster of cells. The inner group of cells become the embryo that eventually becomes a fetus that eventually becomes an earth-side baby.

Conception is a perfect science. That's at once reassuring and daunting. If the brain and body intuitively know what to do, there's nothing left for us to think about, other than what time of the month to have sex. But what if the brain or the body are off-kilter? What if you want to have a child on your own? What if you have an illness or take medications that threaten your ability to naturally conceive or safely carry a baby? What if you want a baby with someone of the same sex? What if? Then what? Then modern science has to replicate what biology does instinctively.

In the summer of 1978, the English town of Oldham was on watch. News crews from around the world had descended on the general hospital, hoping for a glimpse of an elusive expectant mother whose due date had been kept under wraps. The paparazzi was accused of orchestrating a bomb threat to force the woman to evacuate and make an appearance.

London's *Daily Mail* had a leg up, having negotiated exclusive access to the soon-to-be parents, Lesley and John Brown. The couple had been trying to conceive for the better part of a decade, but Lesley's fallopian tubes were blocked and John's sperm couldn't reach her egg. It wasn't going to happen the old-fashioned way.

At the time, though, there wasn't a new-fashioned way. Doctors around the world had performed egg retrievals and had fertilized ovum with sperm, but the resulting embryo transfers hadn't resulted in viable pregnancies. The Browns and their pioneering medical team—namely obstetrician and gynecologist Patrick Steptoe, physiologist Robert Edwards and embryologist Jean Purdy—were about to change that.

On the night of July 25, 1978, Brown delivered a baby girl, Louise Joy Brown, her middle name given for the happiness her existence would bring to those who struggled with infertility. "And here she is . . . The Lovely Louise," the *Daily Mail* announced on its front page. "Louise Brown has chubby cheeks, tiny fists, a mop of unruly blond hair, a voracious appetite and powerful lungs that bellow down the hospital corridor," the story read. The media heralded Louise as a "miracle baby" and "the baby of the century."

It wasn't all celebration though. Debate erupted about the moral, ethical and legal implications of starting life in a laboratory. Religious groups were horrified at the thought of people "playing God" with reproduction. The Catholic cardinal who went on to become Pope John Paul I expressed concern about separating procreation from the act of sex between husband and wife. "Even if the possibility of having children in vitro does not bring about disaster, it at least poses some enormous risks," he was quoted as saying. "Given the hunger for money and the lack of moral scruples today, won't there be the danger that a new industry will arise—that of 'baby-manufacturing,' perhaps, for those who cannot or will not contract a valid marriage? If this were to happen, wouldn't it be a great setback instead of progress for the family and for society?"

The Vatican's thinking hasn't materially changed since then. In May 2023, the Holy See Press Office released a paper urging Catholics not to resign themselves to the "decline of the family in the name of uncertainty, individualism and consumerism, which envision a future of individuals who think only of themselves." The document, known as the Family Global Compact, is aimed at promoting the Catholic Church's vision of family. It stresses the importance of the "man-woman couple relationship." The Church urges couples grappling with infertility to adopt a child or to pursue "naprotechnologies" (natural procreation technologies). It laments, "'a healthy child only at the right time' is now the most common attitude, especially in more advanced countries where technology is most available." Given the Church's stance, I was surprised to learn that one of the world's first fertility drugs—Pergonal, which helps stimulate ovulation and has been discontinued under that name—was developed with the help of hundreds of postmenopausal nuns who donated their urine for research, with the blessing of the Pope.

Louise Brown's birth summoned fears within the medical community, too. "The potential for misadventure is unlimited," Dr. John Marshall, at the time the head of obstetrics and gynecology at Los Angeles County's Harbor General Hospital, told *Time* magazine. "What if we got an otherwise perfectly formed individual that was a cyclops? Who is responsible? The parents? The doctor? Is the government obliged to take care of it?" British geneticist Robert J. Berry told the magazine: "We're on a slippery slope."

I reached out to Louise Brown in the hopes of speaking with her about life as the world's first IVF baby. I wanted to know when and how she learned her birth was historic. I wanted to know whether that realization was profound. I wanted to know what her late parents thought about the IVF process. Brown agreed to respond to my questions via email. She explained that her mother had spent a decade longing for a child. "She would have done absolutely anything to have a baby," she wrote. "That feeling is the same for millions of men and women around the world today. My mum would never say that she was brave, but she was certainly determined and willing to go further than some other people to achieve her dream."

The sentiment Brown went on to describe is one that so many going through infertility can relate to: "My mum and dad had been told they only had a million to one chance of having a baby; my mum heard that as 'there is a chance' and she just followed opportunities."

That fortitude brought her to the medical team in Oldham, though she didn't realize until very late in the pregnancy that her baby would be the first in the world born via IVF, Brown said. Indeed, the case raised serious concerns about informed consent. "They then had to face an incredible media spotlight, hate-mail and being in the public eye," she said. "My mum hated all of that, but she was willing to put up with it to have her baby." Louise would later gain a sister, also by IVF.

Brown said she was four years old when her parents sat her down to talk to her about how she was conceived. Together, they watched a video of her birth. "They told me that they needed help in bringing me into the world from the doctors," she said. "I'm not sure I fully understood it all at that time, but they wanted me to have some understanding before I went to school, as they felt sure people would mention it to me." She knew from a young age that there was something special about her birth, but it wasn't until she was a teenager that she fully realized the significance of it. "By the time I did sex education, I was in the textbooks," she said.

She described feeling proud to have been the first baby born via IVF and said she is happy to spread the word about her parents' pioneering medical team. Dr. Edwards was awarded the Nobel Prize in Physiology or Medicine in 2010. (The other key members of the team, Steptoe and Purdy, were ineligible because they had passed away and the prize is not awarded posthumously.) "Their work," she said, "has brought happiness to millions of people across the world."

Each year in the United States, there are upward of 100,000 live births from assisted reproductive technologies. While still relatively rare, accounting for about 3 percent of all infants born annually in the country, the use of fertility treatments in the United States has more than doubled over the past decade or so. In Canada, there were

8,870 live births resulting from assisted reproductive technologies in 2024, up from approximately 6,000 a decade prior.

Globally, at least twelve million babies have been born via assisted reproductive technologies since that day in Oldham. In the intervening years, fertility medicine has made some significant strides. Medications have become more effective. Fertilization techniques have improved. Vitrification has dramatically reduced damage to embryos during the cryopreservation and thawing process. At its core, though, the IVF process remains largely unchanged. It can be done using a couple's own eggs and sperm to create embryos, or it can be done using gametes from a known or unknown donor. The patient or a surrogate may carry the pregnancy. A treatment cycle—from egg retrieval to fertilization and embryo transfer—can take as little as a few weeks.

A typical round of treatment starts with stimulation of the ovaries and cycle monitoring. A patient calls the fertility clinic to report the first day of their period, known as day one. The first day of a period is considered the outset of the menstrual cycle and marks the beginning of the treatment cycle. Patients go to the clinic for their baseline bloodwork and transvaginal ultrasound around day three of their cycle. A nurse then reviews the bloodwork and ultrasound results with the fertility doctor to confirm the medication protocol. The patient is told which drugs to start, at what dose, at what time and at what frequency. The patient typically goes to the clinic every second day, and then every single day, until the retrieval. Doctors track the reproductive system's response to the hormones and the follicle-stimulating medications they prescribed, tweaking the drugs and adding in new ones along the way.

When not in an IVF cycle, follicle stimulating hormone (FSH) and luteinizing hormone (LH) are naturally secreted from the brain, telling the ovarian follicles to recruit a cohort of eggs to begin maturing. A surge in LH tells the lead follicle to release the dominant egg for the potential of natural conception. You only need one good egg to get pregnant from sex. In IVF, though, the goal is to recruit more eggs than are naturally called to action and to rescue as many eggs as possible. To do that, doctors prescribe pharmaceutically derived FSH, which, when injected into the body, stimulates follicles to mature at a higher rate than normal. Doctors may also prescribe a naturally occurring source of LH, which in the follicular phase of a menstrual cycle recruits more of the FSH receptors in the follicles, making them more receptive to the FSH injection.

A patient's ability to grow follicles depends in large part on the level of anti-Mullerian hormone (AMH) their ovaries produce. The AMH level gives a good indication of how many eggs are in a patient's ovarian reserve. AMH is also considered a proxy for egg quality. The lower the AMH, the more likely it is that the patient will have trouble conceiving. If you're doing IVF, a higher AMH is generally correlated with better embryo outcomes. The more mature eggs you get, the more embryos you're likely to make. The more embryos you make, the more genetically balanced embryos you're likely to have. The more genetically balanced embryos you have, the more likely you are to have one or more viable pregnancies.

Patients are put on one of a handful of ovarian stimulation protocols, usually for somewhere between ten to twelve days. These protocols include a gonadotropin, which is a drug that stimulates follicle growth. Dr. Tamara Abraham, a reproductive endocrinologist at Ontario's Generation Fertility, explained to me how stim cycles typically work. The hormones, which are usually injected into the fat of the stomach, travel through the bloodstream to their target organ, in this case the ovaries. Like interlocking Lego pieces, receptors in the ovaries connect with the hormones, triggering a signal in the cells that tells the eggs to start growing and maturing. Mature eggs are the goal. Why? Because they're more likely to have the correct number of chromosomes and genetic material required to be properly fertilized with sperm.

Ovarian stimulation is a dance. An art and a science, doctors will tell you. You want to grow a nice number of mature eggs, but you don't want too many because that puts you at risk of ovarian hyperstimulation syndrome—a relatively rare but potentially serious complication in which the ovaries swell and blood vessels are unable to retain fluid, causing a detrimental accumulation of fluid in places like the abdomen. You also don't want any of the eggs to become too big. And you definitely don't want to ovulate before your doctor gets the chance to extract the eggs. This is why at a certain point in the stim cycle the patient is told to inject a medication that inhibits the hormone that prompts ovulation. And that's why when the time is right, based on hormone levels and follicle growth, the patient injects a trigger medication to override the inhibitor and cause the body to mature the eggs so they're ready for harvesting. Usually, a retrieval is done thirty-six hours after the trigger shot.

During a retrieval, the patient is typically put under conscious sedation, which is a form of anesthesia that includes a sedative and a pain blocker. A speculum is placed into the vagina. The cervix and vagina are cleaned with a saline solution, and a local anesthetic is injected into the cervix. An ultrasound probe, equipped with a needle-guide attachment, is inserted into the vagina. The doctor inserts a retrieval needle into the guide. The needle can then be inserted through the vaginal wall and into each follicle. The follicular fluid is aspirated out of each follicle and into individual test tubes. Once all the follicles have been aspirated, the retrieval is considered complete. Most retrievals glean between eight and twelve mature eggs. The ideal range is between fifteen and twenty. Some women with low AMH levels are lucky if they produce even a couple mature eggs. The procedure takes about a half hour.

The test tubes are passed to the lab, where an embryologist transfers the fluid to a petri dish and looks through a microscope in search of eggs. The eggs are about 135 microns in diameter, or 0.01 millimetres—not even the width of a hair. They're each surrounded by cumulous cells, which function as their support system. Using a tiny pipette, the embryologist picks up the egg and its surrounding cells and places them into a clean culture medium, which is essentially a complex salt solution with vitamins and amino acids meant to mimic what's in the body.

The eggs are put into a small incubator set to body temperature, or 37 degrees Celsius. What happens next depends on whether the patient is doing conventional IVF or intracytoplasmic sperm injection (ICSI, pronounced ick-see). ICSI is increasingly becoming the fertilization approach of choice and is particularly useful in cases involving issues with the sperm. These days, it accounts for approximately 70 percent of all fertility cycles in Europe, the United States and Canada. Both approaches require sperm, which is provided by a patient's partner or a donor. The semen is typically sent through a centrifuge and then washed through a filter system. A good sample has millions and millions of moving sperm. In some of the most challenging cases of male-factor infertility, there might be one or two moving sperm, or none at all. In those instances, the doctor may perform a testicular retrieval to extract sperm directly.

In conventional IVF, the embryologist uses a pipette to add tens of thousands of sperm to the petri dish containing the eggs, which still have their support system of cumulous cells. Sixteen to eighteen hours later, the embryologist looks under a microscope to see how many of the eggs have been fertilized. As Denny Sakkas, the chief scientific officer at Boston IVF, explained, you "put the sperm in, and they work it out themselves." With ICSI, on the other hand, the sperm don't duke it out the same way. After stripping away the cumulous cells to isolate the egg, the embryologist uses a very fine needle to catch a sperm and inject it into the egg.

The following day, which is considered day one of the fertilization process (not to be confused with day one of the patient's cycle, when their period starts), the embryologist checks to see if any of the eggs have been fertilized. Depending on a number of factors, a patient can expect somewhere between 60 to 80 percent of the mature eggs to fertilize normally. Over the course of the next few days, the embryologist keeps a close eye on the development of the embryos and watches the rate of cell division. By day five, a healthy embryo has formed a fluid sac in the middle of the ball of cells. One group of cells (the inner cell mass) will form the fetus, and another (the trophectoderm) will form the placenta, which passes critical nutrients to the developing embryo. At this point, the embryo is considered a blastocyst and starts expanding. Somewhere between 40 and 60 percent of fertilized eggs make it to the blastocyst stage.

Embryos slated to be frozen for future use are typically cryopreserved between days five and seven of their development. To guard against damage during the freezing process, the embryologist passes the embryos through solutions that effectively suck water from the cells. Otherwise, the water freezes into sharp crystals that could hinder development. The embryologist replaces the water with a cryoprotectant—embryo antifreeze, if you will. The embryos are then flash-frozen with liquid nitrogen, at a temperature of roughly -190 degrees Celsius. They're placed in small tubes or straws in storage containers.

If a patient has opted to do pre-implantation genetic testing, the embryologist biopsies the embryo before freezing it and sends the cells to a specialized lab for analysis. Separate from the genetic testing, the embryos also receive a formal grade, which dictates the order in which they're transferred. The grade is based on several factors, including the rate of expansion and the state of the inner cell mass and trophectoderm.

The attrition rate is real and should be clear to patients. While a number of factors determine the trajectory, this is, generally speaking and on average, how it goes: If a patient retrieves ten mature eggs, they can expect between six to eight to fertilize normally; of those, three or four will make it to blastocyst stage; and of those, maybe two will be genetically balanced.

The next step is a transfer. There are two types of transfers: fresh, in which an embryo is transferred into the uterus a few days after an egg retrieval, and frozen, in which a cryopreserved embryo is thawed and then placed in the womb. In the past, it was thought that fresh embryo transfers were better because the natural environment of the uterus was better at growing embryos than a solution in an incubator. But lab technologies and practices have improved such that frozen cycles generally have equivalent or higher success rates. Increasingly, patients are choosing the frozen route.

Regardless of whether the patient has opted to use a fresh or frozen embryo, the uterine lining must be ready for implantation before a transfer. This requires increased levels of estrogen, whether naturally produced, administered through medication, or both. When the time is right, the patient undergoes a "lining check." An ultrasound technician measures the endometrium's thickness and determines whether it has the trilaminar pattern associated with higher implantation rates. If the lining looks receptive, a patient typically starts taking progesterone. Normally, a transfer takes place on the sixth day of progesterone, though timing can vary slightly.

When it comes time for a transfer, the doctor inserts a catheter into the vagina, through the cervix and into the opening of the cavity of the uterus. The patient is awake. The catheter has room for another catheter to be inserted inside. An embryologist loads the inner catheter with an embryo, and then, under ultrasound guidance, the doctor moves the inner catheter through the outer catheter and into the uterus. Because an embryo is microscopic and imperceptible on an ultrasound, the embryologist loads air bubbles into the catheter along with the embryo so the doctor can see where the embryo is placed based on where the air bubbles are released.

Bloodwork is typically scheduled for nine days after a transfer to determine if it resulted in a pregnancy. The hope, of course, is that hCG is detected. The hope is for what the trying-to-conceive community calls a BFP—a big fat positive.

Medically Necessary

From: Dan Baum
Sent: Wednesday, October 16, 2019, 5:09 p.m.
To: Tom Hannam
Cc: Kathryn Blaze Baum
Subject: Time to meet / guidance on next step?

Hi Tom,
Hope this finds you well . . . I have a few friends who are going through various processes with Hannam, and they've been very impressed/ pleased. Similarly, I was very impressed with you and your clinic when we met a few years ago (albeit under different pretenses), so wanted to reach out.

My wife, Kathryn, and I are thinking about starting the IVF process. We have a 21-month-old daughter, Sidney, who was conceived naturally, but we've had some miscarriage troubles along the way.

For background, in case helpful: we had one miscarriage, at six weeks (cause unknown), before Sidney was born, and have had two miscarriages since she was born—once in April of this year, requiring a D&C at 8/9 weeks (cause was triploidy with the extra chromosomes coming from the egg), and once just this past week, at around six weeks (cause unknown). We'd like to understand what options are available to us and potentially get the ball rolling on IVF. We're both 35 and not getting any younger. We also may want to have a third child, and don't want aging reproductive systems to be the obstacle.

Can you please advise on the right next step? I know you're busy, but any chance you're available to meet with us in the next week or two?

Thanks in advance for your help. Look forward to hopefully chatting with you again soon.

Dan

It had been barely twenty-four hours since we learned we were having another loss, and we were emailing a fertility clinic about potentially starting IVF. We knew, at least intellectually, that IVF wouldn't guarantee success, but we also knew we couldn't stay the course of trying naturally. The definition of insanity is doing the same thing over and over again and expecting different results. We felt like we were going insane.

By this point, we'd had three miscarriages—one before Sid and two after. Something had to be awry. It seemed like more than just bad luck. I look back on the decision to proceed with IVF and wonder if we would have gotten to a viable pregnancy quicker if we'd stuck to trying naturally. It wouldn't have been ill-advised for us to do so. Due to the cost of fertility treatment, most people, unfortunately, wonder the opposite: *If we could have afforded IVF, would we have had a baby sooner? Would we have had a baby, period?* Dan and I were lucky to be considering treatment at Hannam. We were fortunate we could afford an IVF shit-kicking. It was a privilege. We're a dual-income household. Our family was able to help us.

Many clinics charge on a pay-as-you-go basis, invoicing for each aspect of treatment as it arises. Some clinics also offer a bundle or package option for a patient to pay a lump sum for IVF services that they may or may not end up needing. The most expensive payment plans may come with a money-back guarantee if your treatment isn't "successful." Success is defined differently by each plan: It could mean a pregnancy, making it through the first trimester, having a live birth or going home with a baby.

"Welcome to the fertility casino, which frequently presents the rarest of scenarios: A commercial entity offers a potentially money-losing proposition to customers in exchange for a generous supply of in vitro fertilization procedures," reads a 2017 *The New York Times* article on the rise of such cost structures in the space. "People pay tens of thousands of dollars for the privilege, and when they come out with a newborn in their arms they're often thrilled to be on the losing end financially."

To hedge their bets, clinics often restrict access to their guaranteed programs to those more likely to be successful (for example, those who are under a specific age, have promising hormone levels, have a BMI within a certain range and haven't experienced a miscarriage or failed IVF cycle). Inflection, a menopause and family-building education platform, did the hard work of surveying more than three hundred fertility patients involved in these kinds of refund programs and interviewed clinics and third-party plan administrators. The survey showed that about two-thirds of patients succeeded on their first retrieval. That's about double the national average. This is likely because the screening process ensures only "good" IVF candidates are enrolled in the program. "In short, if your clinic has a refund program and offers it to you, this may be a sign they are ultra-confident in your case, and so you may not want to enroll in their program," the platform says.

No matter the payment plan, IVF remains out of reach for many. And while Canada is renowned for its universal health-care system, an exception to this public provision of care is fertility treatment. In general, the provinces and territories, which are responsible for providing health care to their residents, have decided that most fertility treatments shouldn't be considered "medically necessary," so these treatments don't fall into the traditional bucket of publicly insured services.

No province or territory fully covers the costs of fertility treatment. That being said, most offer financial support for IVF and surrogacy through capped funding programs or tax credits. Ontario offers a relatively generous funding program, though advocates say the program is flawed. In 2015, the province announced it would provide patients under the age of forty-three with a paid IVF cycle once per lifetime, as well as unlimited rounds of intrauterine insemination (IUI). (The age threshold was selected somewhat arbitrarily, as there's no globally agreed upon upper limit for undergoing IVF.) The funding program also includes freezing sperm or eggs in cases of medical need, for example ahead of cancer treatment. The program does not, however, cover fertility medications, nor does it cover embryo freezing, sperm washing for IUI or genetic testing. It's not needs-based, meaning people can apply for a funded cycle regardless of their income. Fifty clinics were awarded government-subsidized treatment cycles at the time of the announcement.

Patients looking to do a funded cycle are typically put on a months-long waitlist, which is counterintuitive and counterproductive. When it comes to fertility, time is of the essence. In 2025, after much lobbying by patient advocacy groups, the province announced a $250-million investment over three years. The money will expand the program to new clinics and is expected to cut wait times.

Some countries have generous fertility programs, Israel chief among them. Israel funds nearly unlimited access to fertility treatment for citizens, no matter their religion or ethnicity, until they're forty-five years old or have two children. This pronatalist policy is attributed in large part to the Biblical imperative to reproduce and to a desire to replenish the number of Jews in the world after the Holocaust. Israel is considered the IVF capital of the world, with more cycles per adult female than anywhere else. Denmark, too, has a substantial taxpayer-financed fertility program. The Nordic country covers the cost of three IVF cycles for the first child of a woman living in the country, up to the age of forty. Around 9 percent of babies born each year in Denmark are conceived using assisted reproductive technologies, higher than anywhere else in the world. Other European countries, including Finland and Portugal, have no upper age limit for their funding programs. Public funding for fertility care is a tough sell in countries like the United States. Most Americans depend on employer-provided private insurance plans, which may or may not cover some portion of fertility treatment.

While it's still true that most employers in Canada don't provide significant fertility benefits, things are changing. Canada's big-five banks and technology companies such as Google, Apple, Meta and Snap have upped their funding. In many industries, though, massive gaps in financial support remain. Even if some employers offer coverage for fertility medications through their drug plans, they often provide nothing in the way of financial support for the actual procedures.

The bottom line is that many people need at least some amount of disposable income—and in many cases a large amount—to create a baby through assisted reproductive technology. The couple living paycheque to paycheque that becomes eligible for a funded cycle would have to turn it down if they can't come up with the money for meds. Gay men face the exceptionally daunting prospect of not only finding an egg donor and paying for at least one IVF cycle but also finding a surrogate and paying all the costs and fees associated with a surrogacy journey. "Fertility has become a privatized commodity for the wealthy," said Carolynn Dubé, the executive director of Fertility Matters Canada, a national advocacy organization. "It has become health care for those who can afford it."

And it's heartbreaking. I spoke with an Ontario nanny who tried for years to conceive naturally. When that didn't work, she turned to intrauterine insemination, which also failed, despite numerous attempts. Unable to pay for an IVF round out of pocket, she waited for a funded cycle to become available. When it did, she hoped and prayed and hoped some more that a retrieval would result in embryos and that a transfer would stick. After shelling out several thousand dollars for medication, she ended up with one embryo. Devastatingly, the embryo didn't implant. Her one shot at IVF had failed. There was nothing left to do but keep trying naturally, all while taking care of other people's children, other people's babies.

She is far from alone. This is why organizations such as the Modern Miracle Foundation exist. Co-founded in 2022 by sisters Danna and Randi Grunberg and their husbands, Vlad Amurjuev and McKenzie Scott, the Canadian charity offers applicants grants toward the cost of an IVF cycle. And it's working. The organization has welcomed several Modern Miracle babies.

The sisters know the struggle intimately. Danna experienced two miscarriages, including an exceedingly rare molar pregnancy, in which two sperm manage to fertilize one egg. The miscarriage prompted her to get some basic testing done. At age thirty-one, she discovered that her ovarian reserve was low, especially for her age. After multiple rounds of IVF, she welcomed her first child in 2020. Randi, for her part, was a teenager when she learned she had a medical condition that would prevent her from carrying a child. If she and her husband wanted to have children using their own gametes, they would need to do IVF and find a surrogate. They managed to welcome two children, one in 2022 and another in 2024.

"I remember staring at our baby and thinking, 'How could we help others have this feeling?'" Danna told me. With that, an idea was born. The charity accepted its first round of applications in January 2023, fielding dozens of requests from across Canada. Applicants must provide information from their fertility doctor that includes their probability of successfully conceiving through IVF. That information is reviewed and vetted by a medical board. Because it's a needs-based grant, applicants also provide detailed financial information. Some applicants are single women; most are couples. The organization is funded by donations and by proceeds from a children's clothing line the sisters launched, Mini Mod. The brand's tagline? Infertility sucks.

I spoke with the sisters about how they think about who the grant should go to. "We want to give everybody a chance, but unfortunately we have limited funds so we have to make difficult decisions," Randi said. "We look at the applicant's financial situation, their medical prognosis and their personal story. We spend a lot of time looking through the applications."

Among those who have received a Modern Miracle grant is Jasmin. When I spoke with the Vancouver Island woman, she was thirty-eight years old and twenty-seven weeks pregnant after enduring more than three years of fertility torture. Jasmin, a self-employed occupational therapist, and her partner, Andrew, an operations manager for a non-profit organization, started trying for a baby in the summer of 2020. "He was fine either way about having kids, but I had always known I wanted to be a mom," she said. This kind of dynamic in a couple is one thing when they're trying naturally. It's quite another when they consciously decide to spend thousands of dollars and months or years on end trying to make a baby that only one of them wants more than anything.

"It put a lot of strain on our relationship because I always wanted to keep going, and he was like, 'How much more money are we going to spend on this? And how long are we going to do this for?'" Jasmin said. "That was a big sticking point. He was okay if it didn't work. I wasn't."

In early 2023, after months of trying naturally, several IUIs and an early miscarriage, the couple agreed to pursue IVF with the financial support of Andrew's parents. At the time, there was no provincial funding for IVF in British Columbia, and neither Jasmin nor Andrew had any significant fertility-related medical benefits to speak of. They had put off having a wedding in order to pay for fertility treatment. Their first cycle started off promisingly: four blastocysts to send off for genetic testing. When the results came in, the couple was in shock. All four embryos were abnormal. "I just didn't know that would be an option," Jasmin said through tears. "I thought we would get a couple good ones. I didn't realize it was possible for us to get none . . . Then my mind went to 'Oh shit, is Andrew going to agree to do this again if we're paying it all ourselves next time?'"

They went back to trying naturally for a few months, and every time Jasmin got her period, it was the same conversation: "I'd bring up the topic of IVF . . . I'd ask, 'Are you saying you don't want kids? Because maybe I need to do this on my own.' And he would say, 'I just want to *be* with you.' And I would say, 'I just want to *do this* with you.'" In the fall of 2023, they did a second round of IVF with a $6,000 grant from Modern Miracle. It made a world of difference in the couple's relationship, easing some of the financial pressure. They tried a slightly different protocol that was supposed to help with egg quality, given the genetic results the prior round. Instead, the doctor retrieved just three eggs because Jasmin prematurely ovulated several others before they could be extracted. All three eggs fertilized and made it to day three. Not a single one, though, made it to day six. Another IVF round that gleaned zero genetically balanced embryos.

"People who haven't done IVF think the hardest part is injecting yourself," Jasmin said. "It's not. It's the disappointment. My whole life, if I just worked hard enough, I could get what I was after. I could work really hard and make it happen. This was different."

Several weeks after receiving the brutal news of their second round, the couple received a call from their doctor. What they heard was jaw-dropping: The culture their embryos had been growing in was part of a massive recall. It was toxic. Their embryos had had no chance. "It was weird, but it was almost a relief, because I thought, 'At least it's not us that was the problem,'" she said. The clinic offered the couple the opportunity to redo the cycle, which they did in early 2024. That retrieval resulted in the creation of five embryos. This time, the couple opted to forgo genetic testing. They had lost faith in the process and didn't trust the results would be accurate.

Jasmin did her first transfer in April 2024. It stuck. "I had always fantasized about how I'd tell Andrew I was pregnant," she told me, "but it ended up being me running out of the bathroom in my undies holding a test, asking, 'Is this a line?! Is this a line?!'" After all that time and money—$59,000 in medical expenses, including the money from Andrew's parents and the Modern Miracle grant—the couple had a baby girl in January 2025.

I called Jasmin when her daughter was about two months old. She was out for a walk, wearing her baby in a carrier. I asked her what it was like to be out the other side. "When I was pregnant, someone asked me, 'What's the first thing you want to say to your baby?'" she recalled, overcome with tears of gratitude. "I said, 'I just want to tell her that I've waited so long to meet her.'"

The day after we sent our email to Dr. Hannam about potentially starting IVF at his clinic, he responded with a note saying he was sorry to hear about our circumstances but was hopeful he could help. To determine if we would be good candidates for IVF, we had to investigate five key parameters: eggs, sperm, fallopian tubes, uterus and overall health. Primarily, though, success in IVF comes down to two key predictors: ovarian reserve and sperm count. The former can be measured in a few ways; the most accurate is a blood test that, in the simplest terms, predicts how many eggs a person could grow in a single retrieval cycle. The latter involves analyzing a sperm sample, with a focus on the total motile count—the number of sperm that are moving well. We were on board with undergoing these initial tests, so the Hannam Fertility Centre administration team sent along the patient questionnaires and a welcome sheet. It was among the first of more than four thousand emails we would receive or send about the creation of a baby.

The welcome sheet said one of the clinic's goals was to "see all of our patients pregnant within nine months." I'm sure that was meant to be reassuring, but at the time, it sounded like an eternity to me. I also took it very much to heart. In my mind, it was entirely realistic to think I'd have a little bump the following year.

With the test results, we were off to a solid start. Dan's sperm looked good, and my ovarian reserve was great for a woman my age. "Kathryn, your AMH from 30 October 2019 was 20 picomoles per litre," Dr. Hannam wrote in an email. "An ideal treatment cycle results in 15 to 25 eggs, the exact range that your AMH would predict. Kathryn and Daniel, if you are emotionally ready for IVF, these results could not be better. And regardless of treatment type, we can feel confident that you have enough eggs to build the family you want."

Confident. The family we want. I realize now that while these words buoyed us, they did us the supreme disservice of providing a false sense of certainty. We held onto those words as if they were gospel. When I spoke with Dr. Hannam about this years later, he conceded that his optimism at the outset of our case backfired. "You had an insanely good prognosis," he told me. "I'm playing the odds. And so, as your doctor, I reflect back positivity. You're an example of an instance where that positivity can actually be very hurtful in the end. Had we known then what we know now, it would have been helpful to temper those expectations." Still, he doubled down: "If it's a good prognosis, then I believe we have to be brave enough to say that to you."

I now realize how common it is for patients to have outsized confidence at the starting line. Most are flying blind. We don't know what we don't know. To boot, most patients go into the process with a baseline level of anxiety (and possibly depression) that only intensifies as time goes on. This is precisely why we defer to our doctors. They're the experts. This is what they do, day in and day out. We put our chances of having a baby in their hands. We trust them. We believe them when they tell us they're confident we'll have a child. We don't ask enough questions, and if we do, we don't necessarily listen to responses, or worse yet, we hear what we want to hear. And we don't realize, at least at the outset, that different doctors might give us vastly different advice on how to proceed.

When we started treatment, I thought IVF success rates were much higher than they are. It's not helpful to know the average success rate in the average patient, because that metric is meaningless to the patient at hand. It says nothing of someone's personal chances. But broadly speaking, it's abnormal for a patient to emerge victorious from an IVF cycle on their first try. Even in favourable situations, most first cycles are unsuccessful. People need to know this. A lot of the success comes down to avoiding "treatment drop-out." As Dr. Said Daneshmand, a San Diego–based reproductive endocrinologist who consulted on our case, told me, "For many patients, it's not a smooth journey."

The journey is also complicated by the fact that no two individuals navigate difficult situations the exact same way. They feel differently, they process and grieve differently, they cope differently. That dissonance can tear couples apart. "A lot of the success in fertility treatment comes down to the capacity of the individual or couple to tolerate the inherent disappointments of it," Dr. Evan

Taerk, a reproductive endocrinologist and founding doctor at Toronto's Pollin Fertility told me.

Many people have heard that a woman's fertility drops off at age thirty-five. It sounds hyperbolic, but there's evidence to support that line of thinking. While it's true that a woman's fertility starts to decline around age twenty-eight, the dip is so imperceptible that no doctor cites that age as a real benchmark in family planning. Above age thirty-five, though, the rate of miscarriage and the time to a live birth increases in a meaningful way. "Things start to get very serious from around age thirty-eight or over," Dr. Hannam explained to me. "You can't really promise yourself or anyone that it's going to be okay, that they'll be having a baby with their own eggs after thirty-eight." The average age where "it just won't happen," he said, is forty-two, but "well before that, it's just not as easy."

Fertility patient after fertility patient told me that from their very first appointment, they coasted through decisions while clutching tightly to the core belief that their doctors knew best and would get them pregnant. IVF was a panacea that would solve their problems. An egg retrieval equalled mature eggs. Mature eggs equalled embryos. An embryo transfer equalled pregnancy. An IVF pregnancy equalled a baby. As I did, they looked back at their younger selves with frustration: Why didn't I ask more questions? Why did I let myself go into this whole thing with so much unbridled optimism?

Many people I spoke with felt a similar sense of frustration at their doctors: Why did they give me the impression this would be straightforward? "The takeaway from my first appointment that still sits with me to this day is, 'This will be easy, we're going to get you pregnant,'" one fertility patient told me. "In my mind, it was a guarantee. I was so naive. But how are we supposed to know any better?" Another woman said, "The doctor told me I had the ovaries of a teenager and all would be well, that I should just come back to him when I was ready to get pregnant."

Never in my life had I considered my AMH. Most people don't. This, to me, is a big problem. A significant, unnecessary blind spot. For about $75, a simple AMH blood test can provide critical information about a patient's fertility. A low value is associated with a low ovarian reserve and, likely, low egg quality. With fewer follicles recruited in the lead-up to ovulation, it's less likely that a mature and healthy egg will be released. Low AMH can make getting or staying pregnant difficult. An abnormally high value is associated with polycystic ovary syndrome (PCOS), a common hormone problem that can affect fertility. Those with PCOS may not ovulate naturally. In my perfect world, people would get their AMH tested in their early twenties and somewhat regularly thereafter. One woman I spoke with had an AMH of 12 pmol/L in early 2019 when she was thirty-three. Two years later, it had declined to 10.8. Two years after that, at age thirty-seven, it had dropped to 5.8. Family doctors should be discussing this with their patients, who can then get their levels tested if they choose. I also think the concept of AMH and ovarian reserve should be taught in high school.

With an AMH level of 20, the expectation was that I would produce somewhere in the order of twenty mature eggs per retrieval cycle. "IVF will demonstrate the frequency with which you make genetically balanced embryos," Dr. Hannam wrote in a November 12, 2019, clinical note, referring to the fact that we planned to test our embryos for chromosomal abnormalities. "As a sidebar, we will also be able to check endometrial thickness. I mention thickness because I worry that you would be at risk for multiple D&Cs if you had multiple losses, which I think in your case could be clinically significant. I do not want to overstate this worry and would absolutely support you continuing to try naturally if, after discussion, that becomes the right choice for you both."

We didn't register the bit about lining thickness as particularly consequential. It was a sidebar, after all. And nowhere in the note did it say that an issue with endometrial thickness could mean an inability to carry a pregnancy. In our heads, an issue with endometrial thickness, while potentially "clinically significant," could be fixed with some meds or some other intervention. The next day, we sent a note to our nursing team. The tone and punctuation speak volumes about our ignorant optimism. "We're excited that we're going ahead with IVF," we wrote. "See you Monday!"

That week, we signed a thirteen-page consent document to proceed with treatment. There were risks associated with the various medications and procedures, ranging from the relatively innocuous (fatigue, nausea and night sweats) to the more terrifying (kidney failure, injury to organs, infection and, in extremely rare cases, death). The consent document noted that there is no current consensus as to whether the likelihood of certain birth defects or other abnormalities may be increased in children conceived through IVF or ICSI as compared to naturally conceived children. That being said, the document warned that "certain risks may be increased for pregnancies resulting from IVF, including intrauterine growth restriction (IUGR), Caesarean delivery and multiple gestations. In addition, I/we understand that singleton pregnancies conceived via IVF tend to be born slightly earlier than naturally conceived pregnancies."

We didn't think any of these complications would apply to us, or we discounted them because we were so firmly locked in on our goal of having a baby. I wish we had acknowledged the reality that while some complications might be rare, they have to happen to someone.

We also had to consider the future of our future embryos. To that end, we signed a declaration of intent for the "disposition of embryos," which effectively outlined what we wanted to do with our embryos in certain extenuating circumstances. For example, if I died before the embryos were used, they would be awarded to Dan and come under his complete control. Vice versa if Dan died. We decided that if we died simultaneously, we wanted our embryos to be donated for research purposes (as opposed to having them destroyed or donating them to an infertile couple or person for their use).

In addition, we had to sign off on what would happen if we got divorced. Our options were a) donate the embryos for research purposes, b) destroy them or c) effectively let the courts decide. We chose option C. Thankfully, we never had to test how this would shake out. Not everyone is so fortunate. Perhaps the most high-profile dispute about the disposition of embryos involves actress Sofía Vergara and businessman and actor Nick Loeb. The former couple was engaged to be married but split after undergoing IVF and producing embryos. In an op-ed for *The New York Times* in April 2015, Loeb said they had tried to have a child through surrogacy, but the first transfer didn't take and the second ended in a miscarriage. Vergara and Loeb had two female embryos left.

After they broke up, Loeb filed a complaint in California seeking custody of the embryos in order to attempt to bring them to term via surrogacy, despite Vergara's wishes to instead keep the embryos frozen indefinitely. Loeb argued that while they signed a form stating that any embryos they created together could only be brought to life with both of their consent, the document didn't specify what would happen in the event of separation. He laid out his perspective in the op-ed, exploring the question of whether embryos should be defined as life or property and of whose desire should triumph—that of the person wanting to avoid turning the embryo into life, or that of the individual wishing to create a child?

"These are issues that, unlike abortion, have nothing to do with the rights over one's own body, and everything to do with a parent's right to protect the life of his or her unborn child," he wrote. Loeb ended up dropping the case a year later, after Vergara won a ruling that would have forced him to disclose the identities of two women he impregnated who had abortions decades prior. Vergara's legal team argued that given this past, it was hypocritical of Loeb to claim he was pro-life. In a bizarre twist, another suit was filed in the state of Louisiana—where the couple dated and Vergara had shot a movie—with the embryos listed as plaintiffs. It was a tactical move. Louisiana is an anti-abortion state, where embryos are considered to have rights, including the right to life. The judge there, however, threw out the case, stating that the court had no jurisdiction over the embryos, which were described as "citizens of California." The years-long legal saga ended in 2021, when the Los Angeles County Superior Court sided with Vergara and issued a permanent injunction banning Loeb from attempting to bring the embryos to term via surrogacy without Vergara's consent.

Clearly, these decisions should be taken seriously. And not only is this something to consider at the outset of treatment, before creating embryos, but also at the end of the fertility journey, in the event of leftover embryos.

It's a strange thing to consider. Embryos in a freezer, waiting. But if you're done making or growing your family and you don't want any more children, then who and what are they waiting for? It costs roughly $500 to $1,000 annually to store embryos. Depending on the storage plan, some patients renew their agreement each year. When is it time to let them go? For some people, it's not a decision they want to make. The agreement doesn't get renewed, the fee is not paid, and attempts to reach the patient, including by email, phone and snail mail, are unsuccessful. In those cases, the embryos may be considered abandoned.

The United States has been experiencing a rapid rise in the number of abandoned embryos. Of the approximately one million frozen embryos in the United States, somewhere in the order of 100,000 are believed to be abandoned. Dr. Daneshmand, the San Diego fertility doctor, explained that while it may be legal for a fertility centre to dispose of embryos if storage fees haven't been paid, it's still ethically and morally challenging ground. "What if there's a patient who moved to New Zealand and went off the grid?" he said, by way of example. It's nightmarish to think about a patient returning to a clinic to use their embryos, only to learn they had been destroyed. We don't know how long embryos can last in storage tanks, but it's definitely a long time. In 2025, a baby was born to an Ohio couple from an embryo that had been frozen for thirty years.

As early as the 1980s, there were questions about whether the discarding of embryos is comparable to abortion. Four decades later, in 2024, the Alabama Supreme Court weighed in, ruling on appeal that embryos are "unborn children" for the purposes of civil liability under the state's wrongful death statute. As such, discarding embryos was akin to taking a life. The case at hand involved three couples whose embryos were destroyed at a hospital-based IVF clinic. Court filings state that a patient "managed to wander into the Center's fertility clinic through an unsecured doorway. The patient then entered the cryogenic nursery and removed several embryos. The subzero temperatures at which the embryos had been stored free-burned the patient's hand, causing the patient to drop the embryos on the floor, killing them." In its 131-page decision, the court held that the state's wrongful death act applies to all unborn children, including frozen embryos.

"The central question presented in these consolidated appeals, which involve the death of embryos kept in a cryogenic nursery, is whether the [Wrongful Death of a Minor] Act contains an unwritten exception to that rule for extrauterine children—that is, unborn children who are located outside of a biological uterus at the time they are killed," the justices wrote. "Under existing black-letter law the answer to that question is no: the Wrongful Death of a Minor Act applies to all unborn children regardless of their location."

The ruling sent shock waves through the fertility world. If an embryo was considered an unborn child, the potential for a disastrous civil liability suit hung over the doctors and clinics that presided over their creation, storage and use. A chill settled over the state's IVF clinics, with several immediately pausing their services. Gut-wrenchingly, this meant patient's cycles were cancelled.

I'll never forget listening to an episode of *The Daily*—a podcast produced by *The New York Times*—that came out in the wake of the controversial ruling. It featured a woman who was on the verge of doing an embryo transfer only to be told it wasn't happening and it wasn't clear when or if it would happen. Beyond that, it would be difficult, if not impossible, to have her embryos moved to a clinic outside the state so that she could proceed with a transfer elsewhere. Even the embryo transport companies were scared to touch the frozen cells. Effectively, her embryos were being held hostage. They were hers, but she couldn't do anything with them. My throat tightened as I listened to her speak, her frustration and desperation palpable. Here was this woman on the brink of a true shot at finally making her dreams come true, being told no because of something so unexpected, so out of her control, so wild.

Though some providers resumed their services after Alabama lawmakers passed legislation to shield IVF providers from civil liability, the prospect of future legal challenges continues to loom large.

Day One

I TOOK THE elevator to the fifteenth floor and checked in at Hannam. It was a nice clinic, looked new, had a minimalist vibe. There were no corkboards with baby pictures or handwritten thank-you notes praising doctors and nurses for making miracles happen. There was lots of natural light, when there was natural light to be had. One thing I would come to learn about IVF is that the days tend to start early, in darkness.

I went down a hallway and took a seat along a wall of windows overlooking a stretch of Church Street that is now burned into my brain by the number of times I looked down at it. I was told to wait for the nurse to call my name.

It was a chilly morning in late November of 2019, about a month after our most recent loss. I looked around, scanning the room but careful not to make eye contact with the other patients. What if I knew someone? What if someone knew me? I wasn't embarrassed or ashamed to be there. It wasn't that. There was just something comforting and exciting about keeping our new path mostly to ourselves for a little while.

We had only told a few people we were starting IVF: our parents, siblings, a close friend or two. They were all supportive and expressed no real reservations, though my oldest brother did say something along the lines of "We know people who have been through it, and it can be really hard in its own way." I remember acknowledging the sentiment but feeling like it wouldn't be true for us. What hubris. What overconfidence.

Most of the women at the clinic appeared to be roughly my age, somewhere in their thirties. It was quiet. There was little to no chatter among patients. We were all looking at our phones or books or had our eyes cast to the floor. There was lots of yawning, dark circles under eyes and coffees in hand. Some of us were going straight into work after our appointments, so we'd pulled ourselves together for the occasion of getting our blood drawn and having a transvaginal ultrasound. Others were in sweats or leggings. Nothing like starting your day with a poke in the arm and a probe up your hoo-hah.

It was my turn for bloodwork. I went into one of the cubicles, pulled up my sleeve and offered my left arm. I have good veins, I was told. Had no idea. Glad to hear it. I closed my eyes and turned my head away. I'm not particularly squeamish when it comes to needles, but I didn't need to see it going in or the blood coming out. I felt the needle pierce my skin. Inhale. I heard the vials being snapped on and off the tube draining my blood. I exhaled as the needle was removed. "That's a good trick," I thought. "I'll remember that for next time. Inhale on the insertion, exhale on the extraction."

The nurse put a cotton ball and Band-Aid over the prick. Please go wait in the chairs to be called for your ultrasound, I was told. I took a seat again and waited my turn, looking out the window at the cars passing below. It was so dark outside. So fluorescent in the clinic.

Many other women came before me and many more would follow suit, marching along the same trajectory, day in and day out: bloodwork, empty your bladder (or don't, depending on the reason for your imaging and what type of ultrasound you're getting), ultrasound, meet with your nurse, pick up your medications, take the elevator down to start the rest of your day. I wondered how many of them already had a child, like me. How many were there to make their first baby? Had they had miscarriages, like I'd had? Were they at the beginning of their IVF journey, in the middle or at their wit's end? If they were anything like I was, they were consumed not just by a grand vision for the future but also by the minutiae and microtrauma that often comes with trying to conceive. If they were anything like I was, fertility was the white noise of their life.

We were strangers but also connected, linked by a shared goal and a common struggle. Not everyone, though, was there for IVF. There are many less invasive and less expensive fertility interventions. Such treatments are useful to those with relatively straightforward problems to solve. A patient who has issues producing fertile cervical mucous, for example, might opt for intrauterine insemination (IUI). So, too, might someone whose male partner has a low sperm count or poor sperm volume. With IUI, a strong concentration of sperm can be transferred at a precise time in the patient's cycle. If a patient experiences a hormone problem that prevents them from regularly ovulating, such as PCOS, they can take ovarian stimulation medications that could increase the odds of getting pregnant via intercourse. If a patient has endometriosis—an oftentimes painful and underdiagnosed condition in which tissue similar to the uterine lining grows outside the uterus—hormone treatment or surgery may be effective at unlocking fertility. There's no need, in some cases, for full-blown IVF.

We all chose Hannam for one reason or another: location, a particular doctor, reputation, a technology on offer, an opportunity for a publicly funded treatment cycle, a shorter waitlist than elsewhere. The fact that we had a choice of clinics shouldn't be taken for granted.

In some provinces and territories, there's not a single IVF clinic. In others, there's only one. This makes things unimaginably stressful for those who have far to commute, in large part because everything in fertility is so time-dependent—on the start of your period, on hormone levels, on follicle growth, on abstinence windows, on the thickness of your uterine lining. It's hard enough to slot fertility treatment into your daily life when you live fifteen minutes from the clinic, let alone if you have to take time off work and pay to travel for key procedures on dates you can't foresee well in advance.

While there are somewhere in the order of 120 facilities in Canada that offer IUI and cycle monitoring ahead of an egg retrieval, there are only about thirty-five clinics across the country that also do the more complex and specialized work of IVF. We were in Ontario, so we had options. More than half of the country's IVF clinics are in the province. As a result, Ontario is also a hub for surrogacy.

These days, most IVF clinics in Canada and the United States are privately owned, whether by a physician or group of physicians, or by private equity firms. One of the fastest-growing networks on the continent is The Fertility Partners (TFP), with thirty-six clinic locations across North America, most of them in Canada. Launched in 2020, TFP has a presence in six provinces, representing more than 30 percent of the market cycles, as of 2025.

TFP's founder and executive chairman, Andrew Meikle, is a former dentist who had experience rolling up clinics in the dental-care space. In 2011, he started Dentalcorp, a network of dentists and clinics that grew to include somewhere in the order of three hundred partners by the time he sold the company in 2018. "We did a lot of good things," he said. "It wasn't a cold-blooded roll-up. Education. Mentoring young dentists. Sharing ideas and best practices." When he was thinking about where he could apply the same model, fertility jumped out to him. It was an unconsolidated space in the health-care sector, and it mostly involved a private payer, not to mention the projected growth in the industry.

One of the concerns with private equity firms entering the space is that clinics could prioritize growth and share value above all else, cutting corners to reduce costs before eventually selling. Dr. Meikle pushed back against this narrative. "I'm not interested in prettying up a business to sell—it's not our playbook," he said. "I saw an opportunity to improve the patient journey, reduce wait times and increase clinical pregnancy rates. That's what motivated me."

Dr. Hannam is the owner and CEO of Hannam Fertility, which he founded in 2006. Eight years later, the clinic became part of the Colorado Center for Reproductive Medicine (CCRM) network, which has three dozen centres in the United States and Canada. Hannam Fertility gets somewhere in the order of four hundred referrals per month. Dan had toured the facility when he was looking at investing in fertility clinics as a business opportunity. He had been impressed. Two friends of ours who are Type A had researched clinics in the city and chose Hannam. If it was good enough for them, it was good enough for us.

Dr. Hannam prescribed me a retrieval protocol that involved a two-to-one dose of Gonal-F (a common follicle-stimulating drug) to Menopur (a source of luteinizing hormone that, much like the discontinued Pergonal, is derived from the purified urine of post-menopausal women). I was also prescribed dexamethasone, an oral steroid shown to improve the ovarian response. The primary nurse dedicated to our file, a kind and eminently patient woman, had coached me a couple weeks earlier on how to administer the medications. Dan had come to the "teaching appointment" and taken notes while I practised mixing and loading the syringes. I opened the button of my jeans, unzipped them a bit and folded them down so our nurse could help me get a good look at the optimal injection site. Pinched skin, about two inches on either side of the belly button. To get a sense for the resistance I would feel as the needle entered my body, she had me press a needle tip into a squishy blue ball.

Gonal-F is easy. It comes in the form of a prefilled pen that allows you to set the dosage, twist on a fresh needle tip and then press a button to release the medication and inject it. Menopur was trickier. To create a specific dose, I had to mix a powder in one vial with a liquid diluent in another vial. I had to use Q-Caps, which are basically adapters that let you withdraw solutions from a vial without opening the vial. When it comes to taking fertility medications, the stakes feel high—because they are. The timing and the dose of the medications need to be precise. Get it wrong and the cycle could be sabotaged. Waiting for the next day one feels like forever.

At the outset of my first retrieval cycle that morning in November of 2019, I was waiting at the clinic for my baseline ultrasound. "Kathryn B?" a technician said, looking around the waiting room. I'm right here, I motioned, standing up to gather my things. The clinic staff try to preserve some modicum of privacy by not using patients' last names.

I followed the technician into an exam room. She gave me a couple minutes to remove my clothes from the waist down and put on a gown. It was white with little black dots in the shape of what looked like flowers. "Cute," I thought. I climbed onto the exam table, the long sheet of white sanitary paper crinkling as I lay down and looked up at the ceiling. The room was dim. I confirmed my name and date of birth. Any latex allergies? No. Feet in stirrups. Tush to the end of the table. Knees bent. Let them splay open. Relax. Cold touch of the probe. Pressure. Deep breath. A twinge of pain as the technician gets the angle just right. I closed my eyes. I needed to remember why I was there.

The first time I pressed the needle tip into the pinched skin of my stomach, I felt a hit of relief. We weren't on our own anymore. I looked forward to the next dose of medication, feeling one poke closer to retrieval day, one poke closer to an embryo transfer, a pregnancy, a baby. There was also something oddly empowering about the whole thing. I was the boss of the body that had made a habit of disobeying me. Here I was, telling it what to do through the language of hormones. It was exhilarating to feel such a sense of control.

I felt strong. Tough, even. That's why I didn't want to complain much when my ovaries started responding to the follicle-stimulating medications, swelling with each developing egg. I had been told to expect a bit of discomfort. I knew I was lucky to be in a position to do a retrieval out of pocket and so soon after signing on with a clinic. I was also lucky to be responding so well to the meds. I felt like I had no business complaining.

So I would lie quietly on the exam table for every cycle monitoring appointment, feet in stirrups, while the ultrasound technician measured each maturing follicle. They showed up on the screen as little black spots in the ovary, a honeycomb of ink blots on a Rorschach test. The more crowded my ovaries got, the more painful these ultrasounds became. The more angles the technician had to reach with the probe. The more swollen and tender everything felt. To distract myself, I would often watch a reality show on my phone, earbuds in, glancing at the clock on the wall and counting down the minutes till it was over.

By the end of November, there were twenty follicles growing in my right ovary and another eighteen follicles growing in my left. That's a lot, though not all of them would reach maturity. I felt bloated, not just because of all the eggs I was growing but also because the medications cause water retention. I felt tired. So tired.

That was thanks, in large part, to the increasing level of estradiol in my body. Looking back at photos from this time, I wore the fatigue so clearly on my face. I felt terrible, and I wasn't fooling anyone.

When it was time for the retrieval, I was prescribed a dual trigger of Pregnyl, which is a form of hCG believed to be linked to improved egg maturity and successful ovulation at the time of a retrieval, and Lupron, a gonadotropin-releasing hormone agonist that tells the brain to begin the process of releasing the eggs. By this time, my estradiol was above 14,000, which is considered within the desired range for a stimulation cycle, and I had grown forty follicles measuring between 1 and 2.8 centimetres. When estradiol is elevated, when a woman has more than twenty follicles growing and when she is on the thinner side, as I am, the risk of ovarian hyperstimulation syndrome (OHSS) is believed to rise significantly. Looking at my stimulation record, I see that someone wrote r/o OHSS. *Rule out ovarian hyperstimulation syndrome.* In extreme cases, OHSS can result in hospitalization for kidney failure, ovarian torsion, and breathing problems.

At the time of my treatment, patients were routinely prescribed an hCG trigger as a way to all but guarantee they successfully released their eggs—even though this increased their risk of OHSS. The thinking has since changed, Dr. Hannam explained to me years later. These days, he said, doctors will consider forgoing an hCG trigger in favour of a single trigger of a GnRH agonist drug—which by itself is less likely to cause OHSS but is also not guaranteed to work.

When I spoke with Dr. Hannam years later about why my protocol included an hCG trigger shot even though I was vulnerable to OHSS, he said he stood by the decision and noted that he prescribed me a low dose. "You're asking me, 'What would I do today, in 2024, and would it probably be the same?'" he said. "I would do the same thing again." He said my bloodwork and stimulation sheet supported the use of hCG, particularly since people who are on the thinner side tend to have a harder time releasing eggs with the

GnRH trigger alone. Put simply, the benefits outweighed the risks.

My trigger injections were set for 10:30 p.m. and 11:30 p.m. on December 3, 2019, as well as 11:30 a.m. on December 4. I set alarms on my phone and had Dan set alarms, too, in case we fell asleep. My first retrieval, at a cost of around $16,500, including pre-implantation genetic testing but excluding medications, was scheduled for the morning of December 5, 2019. On retrieval day, I was led to the procedure area, which is separate from where the cycle monitoring takes place. It felt good to cross the threshold. I was shown to my own little recovery bay, sectioned off from the nurses' desk with a curtain. I stripped off my clothes and put on a periwinkle-blue medical gown with a matching disposable cap and foot covers. I took a selfie at 8:31 a.m. and sent it to my sister. I can see the hope and innocence in my eyes.

I can see the version of myself that thought this was a silver bullet, that thought she would be pregnant soon. I feel bad for her. She's so naive. So unaware of all the ways this would go sideways, hurt her. Perhaps that was for the best. But I still wish I could go back, take her face in my hands, look her in the eyes and tell her to be patient. To let go of her arbitrary timelines. To let go of looking ahead at the calendar, picturing how big her bump would be for this friend's wedding or that family vacation. I wish I could hug her and tell her it will be a long road but it will be okay.

One of the nurses took my vitals, checking my blood pressure, pulse, temperature and oxygen levels. She then went over the consents with me, explaining the medications I would be given and what would happen in the operating room.

I was given an Ativan, which is a benzodiazepine medication. I put the small white pill under my tongue and let it dissolve, leaving a bitter taste in my mouth. "It will help relax you," the nurse said. Within minutes, I felt a sense of calm wash over me. The Ativan slowed everything down, gave me a full-body deep breath. My mind quieted, and I was at ease. The nurse inserted an IV, which would administer fluids to keep me hydrated throughout the procedure, Gravol to help prevent nausea and an antibiotic to guard against infection.

The Ativan-Gravol combo sent me into the perfect peaceful drowsiness. IV pole in tow, the nurse helped me to the nearby bathroom so I could empty my bladder on the way to the procedure room. A team was inside waiting for me, prepping the necessary medications and instruments. One of the nurses helped me onto the bed. I placed my feet into the stirrups, knees touching to guard my privacy until I had to splay them open. There's no modesty in fertility. There's no room for it. The work can't be done without exposing yourself. Your body is laid out for strangers to see and to know. A certain level of intimacy is required.

I don't remember much of what happened next. I was administered two more drugs for pain management—fentanyl and Versed, which together pulled me into a state known in the medical world as conscious sedation. Colloquially, it's sometimes referred to as "twilight" because it suppresses consciousness without putting the patient all the way to sleep. The procedure room and all the faces around me became foggy, and then I was out. I recall regaining some measure of awareness at one point, feeling pressure in my ovaries, and then lulling back into black. Next thing I knew, I was back in my recovery bay, feeling only slightly more conscious than when I was under conscious sedation. I'm a wuss when it comes to experimenting with drugs, but I loved what I was feeling. I adored emerging from that drug combination. There was something ethereal and serene about floating in the space that exists between asleep and awake.

Dr. Hannam came to my bedside to let me know how the procedure went. Thankfully Dan, who sometime during all this had provided his sperm sample, had come to the recovery area to take in the information. The only thing I recall from this exchange is seeing Dr. Hannam's face. I couldn't absorb any numbers or specifics, but the takeaway was that the retrieval had gone well. I started to get my bearings and was able to get dressed. Dan held my arm as we walked to the elevator and made our way to the car. When we got home, I crawled into bed and closed my eyes.

The notion of discomfort in IVF is entirely subjective. I was told to expect spotting, mild abdominal cramping, bloating and potentially some constipation and gas pain. I was advised to call the clinic or go to the emergency room if I experienced severe abdominal pain not relieved by Tylenol, severe vaginal bleeding that required changing pads at least every two hours or a high fever. To me, this meant anything that didn't reach those thresholds was par for the course, particularly after such a "successful" retrieval that resulted in the aspiration of fifty-three follicles. It seemed like I was supposed to grin and bear it, as if it hurt so good.

The day after the retrieval, we received a call from Hannam's lab with an update on the fertilization. We were told that a total of thirty-one eggs had been extracted. On day one, the day after the retrieval, twenty had been successfully fertilized with Dan's sperm. They all made it to day three. The next significant update would come on day five or six, at which point whichever blastocysts had made it that far would be biopsied for genetic testing and frozen.

A couple of days after the retrieval, a nurse called to check in on me and see how I was feeling. I missed her call because I was having a nap, so I sent an email. "I'm still in discomfort and want to make sure that's 'normal,'" I wrote. It felt like my insides had been . . . not sliced and diced, that's too strong but . . . pierced? Cut? Scraped? I suppose my ovaries felt exactly like what had been done to them. They had been poked by a needle fifty-three times. It hurt to go from standing to sitting. It was hard to take a deep breath. I was exhausted, and my face was swollen and puffy. A nurse called me and explained that fluid may start to leak into the pelvis and abdomen. As a result, my body would lose electrolytes, such as potassium and sodium. I was advised to abide by the hyperstimulation management protocol, which involves consuming lots of fluids and salt. I ate Mr. Noodles in a Cup, pickles and Lipton chicken noodle soup—the neon-yellow kind—pretty much on repeat. I was told to monitor and record my input and output of urine. This meant peeing into measuring cups to make sure that what was going in was coming out. I also started to record my weight and waist measurement daily, to see if things moved in the right direction.

In my discomfort, life went on. We took Sid to a museum to look at a dinosaur exhibit. We baked banana muffins and went out on the sled. Having just transitioned to covering the environment beat for *The Globe*, I filed a story on Volkswagen AG's diesel emissions scandal. I snuck a beaker into the newsroom bathroom and peed into it, taking note of my "output" before spilling the urine down the toilet and returning to my desk. I was at work when the lab called with our final update. It was a good result: Six blastocysts had developed normally and were biopsied for genetic testing. The biopsied cells were sent to CCRM's lab in Colorado, while the embryos themselves were frozen and stored onsite in Toronto.

We opted for pre-implantation genetic testing because our history of pregnancy loss raised questions about our propensity to create balanced embryos. A woman of my age could expect about half of the embryos to be considered chromosomally correct. Of the six we had just made, somewhere in the order of three were expected to be euploid embryos. Pre-implantation genetic testing is good at reducing the rate of miscarriage, though it doesn't remove the risk entirely, since losses can occur for other reasons. It also hasn't been proven to increase the rate of live births across the board.

Human DNA is comprised of twenty-three pairs of chromosomes. Embryos with missing or extra chromosomes are known as aneuploid embryos. Down syndrome, for example, is the most common chromosomal abnormality and is caused by having three copies of chromosome 21. Aneuploidy embryos have less chance of developing into a baby. When a patient opts for genetic testing, biopsied cells are tested and considered representative of the health of the embryo as a whole.

Because older women are more likely to have eggs with missing or extra chromosomes, pre-implantation genetic testing for aneuploidy (PGT-A) isn't considered particularly useful or beneficial to younger patients (those under about thirty-five) who don't have a history of recurrent miscarriage or a family history of chromosome problems. For these women especially, PGT-A could prove an unnecessary expense. It may create an unnecessary delay in the patient's journey, as they wait for genetic results to come back. It could cause damage to the embryo and prevent it from developing upon transfer. In addition, there are instances of misdiagnosis, particularly in cases involving mosaic embryos.

Mosaic embryos contain both euploid and aneuploid cells—that is, both normal and abnormal cells. "The proportion of euploid and aneuploid cells can impact the chance of successful outcome if the embryo is transferred," according to the Human Fertilisation and Embryology Authority, the United Kingdom's independent regulator of fertility treatment and research. "Mosaic embryos may have a lower chance of pregnancy, but there are reports of healthy live births after a transfer of a mosaic embryo." Embryos are either considered low mosaics or high mosaics. Low mosaics have a lower proportion of abnormal cells and therefore are more likely to result in a healthy live birth. "There are concerns that mosaic embryos may be discarded if PGT-A analysis looks at only the portion of cells from the embryo that all happen to be aneuploid, when they also contain normal cells and may be able to result in a live birth," the authority said. One of the women I spoke with had a child from a low-mosaic embryo. "Most people don't use their mosaics," she said. "My perfect little boy is a mosaic." She pointed me to a Facebook page called My Perfect Mosaic Embryo. It has more than twenty-one thousand members.

On December 13, eight days after the retrieval, I sent another email to my Hannam team to let them know I still didn't feel right. I was nowhere near back to myself. We had a work event with Dan's colleagues that evening, so I got myself together and put on a forgiving dress that would hide my bloated tummy. The thought of someone mistaking my post-retrieval bloating for a budding baby bump was a devastating irony. I was self-conscious the entire night. It was self-centred to think anyone was wondering whether I was pregnant, but that's where my mind was.

The next day, I updated the clinic with my waist measurement, which was a couple inches larger than usual. I still couldn't wear most of my pants or skirts, opting instead for stretchy leggings or the jeans I bought when I was seventeen weeks pregnant with Sid or the ones I got when I was three months postpartum. I muscled through those post-retrieval days until slowly but surely, I could feel my body normalize, my hormones level off. Getting my period after a retrieval became a milestone. Once I started my cycle, I felt like myself again. It was as if my uterus wasn't just shedding my lining: It was shedding the burden of that month's IVF treatment. I was starting fresh. Tabula rasa.

When It Rains

THE DAY STARTED with a candle in a stack of pancakes. It was January 17, 2020, Sid's second birthday. It was bittersweet, though in hindsight I wish I'd embraced the sweet and left no room for bitter. I thought for sure I would be pregnant with her brother or sister by this point. But things were looking up. We had done a retrieval, gotten lots of eggs that turned into a good number of embryos. We were waiting for the results of the genetic testing.

So much of fertility treatment is waiting. Waiting to start your period. Waiting to start your injections. Waiting to trigger. Waiting to transfer. Waiting for the lab to call with results. Waiting for the pregnancy test. Waiting in the waiting room. The patience required to get through a day in the life and mind of a fertility patient is extraordinary. So much is out of your control. Time is just one element of that. We can't make the clock spin faster. And if you otherwise love your life, you don't actually want it to; you don't want the days to fly by. I didn't want Sid to get older. I didn't want to wish away her younger years. I didn't want to always be counting down toward something. But that's the resting state of treatment. Counting the days, trying to get to the next step, clamouring for the chance at good news. Perhaps some fertility patients don't feel this way, but I haven't met them.

The genetic results had been delayed, but our nurse had told us that January morning that we would likely be getting a call with the news later in the day. Every time my phone rang, my heart skipped a beat. But the workday came and went without a call from Hannam.

By the time we sat down to Sid's birthday dinner at one of our favourite restaurants, we assumed we wouldn't hear from the clinic that day. I smiled for a photo with Sid as she hoovered buttered penne. We laughed as we watched her try my sparkling water, her face squishing and shoulders shuddering as the bubbles fizzed on her tongue. And then Dan's phone rang.

"Dan speaking," he said. He got quiet, listening. He mouthed "Dr. Hannam" to me. I figured Dr. Hannam was calling with the results of the genetic testing; I also thought it was odd that the call was coming so late and that he would be delivering the news himself, given that so much of our communication thus far had been with our nurse. "How many?" I whispered to Dan. He looked at me and held up his index finger. One. One good embryo out of the six we sent? "One?" I whispered to him. He nodded and then passed me the phone.

I left our table and found a quiet spot near the restroom to speak with Dr. Hannam. He explained that only one of the embryos had come back with the correct number of chromosomes. Another one came back as inconclusive and could be re-biopsied, for a fee. The other four were deemed genetically "incorrect." This, he said, could explain why we'd had so many losses. Maybe we don't tend to make genetically balanced embryos. I was devastated. I knew what this meant. I would probably do another retrieval. We weren't going to use the only good embryo we had, without any backup in case of another miscarriage. And what if we wanted a third child?

There would be no transfer on my next cycle, no potential for a pregnancy in a few weeks. Likely no 2020 baby.

But there was more. On Christmas Eve, I had gotten a sonohysterogram, which provides imaging of the structure of the uterus. It can detect polyps, fibroids and other issues that can complicate getting and staying pregnant. A technician inserted a catheter into my cervix and flushed saline fluid into my uterus, causing some cramping. The sonohysterogram, Dr. Hannam told me, had showed that there was a mid-body adhesion in my uterus, likely from the D&C I'd had the year prior.

An adhesion is scar tissue, he explained. The uterus is supposed to be shaped like an upside-down pear, wider at the top and narrowing at the bottom toward the cervix. In my case, a band of scar tissue connected the two sides of my uterus, causing the right and left sides of my lining to stick together. Instead of looking like a pear, my uterus looked more like an hourglass. The band of scar tissue blocked the saline fluid from reaching the uppermost part of the uterus known as the fundus. Adhesions, he explained, could interfere with implantation and increase the risk of miscarriage. I had what's called Asherman's syndrome.

He advised that I get a consult with a gynecological surgeon to discuss surgery to have the scar tissue released so the two walls could become unstuck. The hysteroscopy procedure would not be without risks, including potentially making the situation worse. I needed to have a discussion with the surgeon and then we could regroup.

I hung up the phone and stood there, outside the restroom, stunned. We thought we'd get a few balanced embryos, or at least a couple. We thought we were doing a transfer next month. We thought we'd have a baby this year. Instead, I needed to do a second retrieval. Another $20,000. For many, that single embryo would have been their one and only shot with IVF, a prospect that would be unbearably nerve-wracking with the newfound knowledge of uterine issues. I also likely needed uterine surgery. And who knew when that could take place. Which should come first, the retrieval or the procedure? Would either be successful?

That phone call changed everything. Our bubble was burst. IVF was not going to be straightforward for us. Tears in my eyes, my head spinning, I made my way back to the table. I explained to Dan what Dr. Hannam had told me. We had already spent more than a year trying to make a baby. We felt like we were so close, on the precipice, and now the goalpost was moving away from us. Dan reached for my hand and squeezed it, knowing I was gutted but putting on a brave face for Sid. The server brought over a bowl of ice cream and we sang "Happy Birthday," my voice shaking with anxiety for what was to come and with gratitude for the child I already had.

We barely slept and woke up the next day to a massive flood in a bathroom, which caused damage to the floors upstairs and on the main level, saturated our kitchen cabinetry, soaked through rugs and ruined some of our furniture. It was clear that we would have to move out, probably for a few months, to remediate and restore our home.

When it rains, it pours.

The flood was pathetic fallacy. We were drowning. You might think, "What's the big deal? You can afford to do more treatment. You have to wait a few more months to make a baby, but that's a child you'll have forever, a sibling for Sid she'll have forever. In the context of your life, this is a blip." That may be true, but a fertility struggle has the horribly powerful ability to strip you of perspective and mess with your concept of time. An hour feels like a day, a day feels like a week, a week feels like a month, a month may as well be an entire year. Each bit of bad news is another tiny cut into an open wound. You don't get to heal from one disappointment before another one is layered on top. The effect is pernicious. I was starting to feel more beat down than hopeful.

Especially as I read more about Asherman's syndrome. Again, I found myself on the National Organization for Rare Diseases website: "Asherman's syndrome is a rare, acquired, gynecological disorder of the uterus. It is characterized by the bonding of scar tissue that lines the walls of the uterus, which decreases the volume of the uterine cavity." *Acquired* means the person is not born with the condition. It may occur as a result of surgical scraping, for example from a D&C, or as a result of an infection of the endometrium or unknown causes.

There aren't any good figures on the prevalence of uterine adhesions. Asherman's tends to lead to lighter periods, but if you're someone who has always had relatively light or normal periods, like me, then you might not clock the decreased flow as unusual or cause for concern. Unless a person loses their period altogether, and unless they investigate their uterus through hysteroscopy or sonohysterogram, they are likely to have no idea they have Asherman's. I myself had no clue. I didn't know this was a thing. While a small percentage of D&Cs overall result in scar tissue, a not insignificant percentage of D&Cs to remove retained tissues of pregnancy are believed to result in adhesions. Some studies put the risk as high as 25 to 30 percent. It was only the start of what I didn't know—about my uterus and about what surgeons would do to it.

With no embryo transfer date in sight, we were in what Dr. Hannam called the "ducks-in-a-row phase." Toward the end of January, I met with a gynecological surgeon and went over the options: go ahead with a hysteroscopy or leave it alone and hope I get pregnant anyhow. I decided to proceed with the surgery. Because the procedure would be done in the public health-care system, I needed to wait for an opening on the surgeon's schedule at a hospital. It was looking like early March, which at the time seemed forever away but in hindsight was quick. In the meantime, I would do another retrieval.

It felt good to use every window of time toward the goal of making embryos and carrying a baby. To Dan and me, there was nothing worse than dead time. I would spend February injecting myself with stimulating medications and doing another retrieval, and I would spend March undergoing a hysteroscopy and healing from it. It seemed reasonable to think we could do a transfer in April or May.

Dr. Hannam tweaked our retrieval plan, recommending ICSI instead of conventional IVF, at an added cost of $1,800. Developed in the early 1990s, ICSI was initially indicated for male-factor infertility cases, in which there are concerns about the concentration, motility (ability to swim forward) and shape of the sperm. But it's become the go-to, regardless of whether there are identifiable issues with the quality or quantity of sperm. Some clinics exclusively offer ICSI, including Dr. Daneshmand's San Diego Fertility Centre.

His view is that ICSI, as a uniform protocol, helps patients bypass potential unforeseen issues that could lead to poor fertilization. He doesn't buy the argument that nature does a better job than science of choosing which sperm should fertilize an egg. "We have developed systems and protocols through research that allow us to overcome the obstacles that nature has imposed," Dr. Daneshmand said. "If you have patients coming to you and spending incredible amounts of resources, you're not going to go back to the 1980s and offer standard IVF."

Even though we had no sperm-related issues, it made sense for us to try ICSI on our second round of fertilization. Conventional insemination hadn't brought the results we'd hoped for. We had gotten a huge number of eggs from the retrieval, but we only ended up with six blastocysts. And of those six blastocysts, only one or two was genetically balanced. Changing things up seemed like a good idea, even if it wasn't clear why our cycle hadn't gleaned the expected results.

At the start of my next period, I called in my day one to begin cycle monitoring for my second retrieval. I knew what to expect this time around. How to mix the medications, what the transvaginal ultrasounds would feel like when my ovaries were full and swollen. Dr. Hannam planned to lower the dose of the hCG trigger, from a half to a quarter dose, but he was prescribing me hCG nonetheless.

The stim days came and went, the same uncomfortable ultrasounds, fatigue and bloating. The retrieval came and went, the same blissful conscious sedation, the same pain in my ovaries in the immediate aftermath. We got thirty-four eggs this time. Of those, nineteen were mature and injected with sperm. Sixteen of them fertilized and made it to day three. By day six, six embryos had progressed normally into blastocysts. We sent them off for genetic testing and began the wait.

The day after the retrieval, a nurse called to check in on me. I told her that I felt rough, similar to the last time but worse. Given what I knew by this point, I wondered if I was experiencing OHSS. I think Dr. Hannam called later that day to check in. Around 9 p.m., he sent an email to our nursing team and me reviewing my symptoms and reassuring me that there was likely no major cause for concern. He offered a plan, saying the team would call daily to check in until there was a resolution. Then he signed off: "Kathryn, you are doing everything right."

If I was doing everything right, why did I feel so horribly wrong? I was confined to my bed, feeling like I had been hit by a truck. My face was puffy, my eyes glassy and set in dark circles, my left eyelid randomly swollen almost shut. I was so bloated I looked pregnant, increasingly so by the hour, it seemed. I was constipated. I had gained several pounds in the couple days since the retrieval. I started to develop shortness of breath and felt light-headed, not to mention the gripping headaches.

I communicated this to Dr. Hannam, who sent another email to my team: "She is having symptoms of OHSS vs. deep discomfort from oversized ovaries," he wrote. He requested that they book me for an ultrasound the following day. "We need to look to either possibility."

When I got to the clinic, our nurse asked how I was feeling and took my vitals. My blood pressure was a bit low. I felt like a slug and looked like hell. An ultrasound confirmed that I had moderate to severe OHSS. More than 1600 ml of free fluid had seeped from my ovaries, some of it into my pelvis and abdomen. This wasn't a case of hyperstim that was likely to resolve itself. I needed to undergo a procedure to drain the biggest pockets of fluid.

I was relieved to hear I wasn't going crazy, that I had good reason to have stayed home from work and lain in bed, sleeping on and off for the better part of four days. Treatment tends to breed doubt—about the process, about your prospects, but also about yourself. I'm supposed to be grateful I have so many follicles. I'm supposed to be a warrior fighting for a child. Why couldn't I see then that I could be a grateful warrior *and* in a concerning amount of pain?

When you do a retrieval, your medical team likely tells you that you'll be able to go to work the next day. That was absolutely not my experience. It would have been helpful to better prepare for the worst, or at least the possible. I realized in that moment that as a woman going through fertility treatment, I needed to listen to my body and trust what it was telling me. No one had properly prepared me for how physically awful this might be. No one told me—really told me—that because I had so many follicles and because I'm petite,

I would almost assuredly be knocked on my ass, my insides crowded with fluid and raging with gas pain. Not all women have as terrible a physical experience as I was having post-retrieval; I should make that clear. I spoke with women who grew a few follicles, and their physical recovery was tolerable. But my expectations, and the expectations of many other women I have spoken with, were not adequately calibrated. I couldn't help but feel blindsided. Some amount of pain and discomfort is par for the course in fertility treatment, but it isn't all inevitable and it isn't all unforeseeable. We can't throw our hands up and say, "That's just part of the deal." Some of it just plain isn't.

The draining procedure took place at Hannam on February 19, 2020. I wasn't under conscious sedation. I was very unwell, fully conscious, legs wide open, instruments inside. I started shaking uncontrollably, tears filling my eyes as I stared at the ceiling. Dr. Hannam told me I was likely quivering because I was nervous about what was happening. Who wouldn't be? My body wasn't my own. It was taken over, overwhelmed.

Dr. Hannam removed enough of the free fluid from enough of the pockets that I would likely feel better in a day or two. My body would be able to handle the rest. Thankfully, it did, but not before I had to cancel a trip to Kelowna to see my family. Dan, Sid and I had been planning to fly out west together, and then Sid and I were slated to stay at my parents' place while Dan joined some friends for a ski trip. I all but forced Dan to go ahead without us. So much of our life had already been interrupted by managing miscarriages and fertility treatment. So many plans—the big things, the little things—had been cancelled or set aside. Treatment robs you of any kind of predictability. It's grating. I'd had enough.

I knew I was in a bad place physically, and I could tell Dan was having trouble emotionally. I could see his optimism being eroded, chipped away at. It was important for him to go, have fun, forget about all this for a weekend. It was important to *me* that he go. It was my way of reclaiming some control. There was no way I could travel, but there was no reason both of us should be held back.

Each day I felt better and better, more and more like myself. I worked from home, still feeling self-conscious about my bloated belly and not up for commuting downtown to the newsroom. By the end of February, I was well enough to moderate a *Globe* panel on the Canadian resource sector in my still relatively new role as environment reporter.

On a chilly early March day, I ran a ten-kilometre race event alongside my youngest brother. I listened to an old running playlist as I jogged, struggling to keep the pace I had grown accustomed to before treatment. But I was proud of myself for putting one foot in front of the other. It had been a while since I'd ran. Fertility patients shouldn't exercise, at least not intensely, during stimulation or until about a week after a retrieval (or until you feel back to normal). That added up to a lot of time spent idle, particularly for someone who relishes in the endorphins released during exercise. I work out as much for my mental health as for my physical health, if not more.

It felt so good to sweat through my fleecy black toque, get rosy-cheeked and out of breath. As I ran along the waterfront, I felt hopeful again. The genetic testing results from the second retrieval had come back, and they were good. Great, even. Of the six embryos we biopsied, four were determined to be genetically balanced. This was a massive win for us. We now had five good-looking embryos—enough to give us some confidence we could likely make two babies, if we wanted. Some women get lucky and it takes only one embryo transfer for them to get pregnant. But in an average IVF case, two or three embryos equals one baby. We felt like we could move on, mentally, from the embryo-making phase. We turned our attention to the next matter at hand: the scar tissue in my uterus, the womb that needed fixing.

A few days later, Dan and I dropped Sid off at daycare and drove to a hospital in the city's east end for the hysteroscopy. I got set up with an IV, trusting yet another team of doctors and nurses with my reproductive health. When I woke up from the general anesthesia, the room was a blur, but I remember the surgeon telling me my uterus had "opened up beautifully."

The plan was to do an embryo transfer the following month. We had already received an estimate for the transfer, $3,350, not including the medications. The plan was to keep moving the ball forward. We were in the end zone. We were so close. But there's an old Yiddish saying: *Mann tracht, un Gott lacht.*

Man plans, and God laughs.

The Long Pause

ON MARCH 11, 2020, about three months after a cluster of patients in Wuhan, China, started to experience symptoms of a pneumonia-like virus, the World Health Organization declared a global pandemic. Already overrun hospitals and health-care systems were increasingly overwhelmed with the new virus, dubbed COVID-19.

It wasn't long before states of emergency were declared in jurisdictions around the world. Schools were shuttered. Flights were grounded. Borders were closed. Doctors and nurses couldn't get their hands on much-needed protective masks and gowns; the demand was too high, the supply chains too logjammed. Life-saving surgeries were cancelled. I don't need to dwell too much here on how hellish the pandemic was. We all lived through it. That being said, our treatment was affected by COVID, so this next part of the story reflects that reality.

My surgeon's office remained open, so I went for my follow-up appointment on March 17, nine days after the hysteroscopy, as planned. I remember leaving the office feeling uneasy about all that was going on around me. The masks, the sanitizer, the closed doors and drawn blinds. But I was also feeling hopeful. I expected my period in about ten days or so, and I couldn't wait to call in my day one for a transfer cycle.

It's hard to overstate the anticipation an IVF patient feels before a transfer cycle. It's the consequential next step, the one that could actually get you pregnant. You do everything you can to optimize the situation. Eat healthy, no alcohol, lots of supplements, prioritize sleep, keep stress at bay. It was absolutely gutting, then, to get an email from Hannam a few days after my post-op appointment, saying the clinic was suspending in-person operations due to the pandemic. For how long? Unclear.

The move was recommended by the Canadian Fertility and Andrology Society. The American Society for Reproductive Medicine as well as the European Society of Human Reproduction and Embryology released similar guidance. The news sent me spiralling into what I now recognize as the five stages of grief. Denial (*Surely this somehow didn't apply to patients who were so close to doing an embryo transfer*). Anger (*Was this seriously happening*). Bargaining (*Maybe another clinic would do a transfer if we moved our embryos*). Depression (*Why was this so hard for us? Was the universe trying to tell us something? Were we destined not to have any more children? I'm so sad*). Acceptance (*I wish I could say I made it to this stage*).

"I'm still in shock that we were at the fucking one-yard line and this is happening," I wrote in an email to a friend. "Yes, I know the world is ending—people are dying and struggling to put food on the table—but this has been our life for the past year. I've taken such a shit-kicking, physically especially, in the past six months. I feel like I've aged five years in five months, just by virtue of the toll on my body of all these procedures and complications. Trying not to feel sorry for myself, but right now, that's where I'm at. We're realizing the best we can do is sit tight and see what the thinking is / options are in a few weeks, when things might be clearer . . ."

My friend's response was reassuring. And prescient. "You're allowed to be selfish and devastated at the moment," she wrote. "And I think also allowed to feel sorry for yourself. At least for a little while. It's going to be okay though. You're going to have another baby. Big picture, twenty years from now, your family is going to look pretty close to how you envisioned it."

The pause in fertility treatment strikes at the core of a much larger debate about whether reproductive health care is on par, in terms of import, with health care in general—whether it's medically necessary, whether access to it should be considered a human right. The World Health Organization says all of its member states have ratified at least one international treaty that includes the right to the highest attainable standard of health. The United Nations' Universal Declaration of Human Rights, which was approved in 1948 by forty-eight countries, including Canada and the United States, recognizes the right to found a family. The right to found a family, though, says nothing of genetic relation or method.

"If we decide it's a person's right to have a child, you have to have a way to exercise that right," said Maureen McTeer, a Canadian lawyer who specializes in medical law and public policy and the author of *Fertility: 40 Years of Change*. "If an infertile couple says it's their right to have a child, do they have a right to commandeer an egg, sperm or a uterus? If the answer to that is that 'No, in such a situation, nobody can commandeer reproductive material or capacity just because someone claims they have a right,' then what? We have to have this kind of discussion so we can resolve these issues."

While the world was ending and ours was on pause, life went on. With Sid home from daycare and Dan also working, we were burning the candle at both ends, as everyone was. I had pivoted to investigating the impact of the pandemic on temporary foreign workers on farms and in meat-packing plants. Many of these people faced poor working and living conditions that defied public-health orders and put them at an increased risk of contracting and spreading the virus. It was hard not to stress about what the stress of my work was doing to my reproductive health, but it was a good distraction and gave me a sense of purpose outside myself. It gave me perspective.

For a while, I didn't tell my editors about our fertility struggle. I didn't want them to think I was distracted from my work. I wasn't sure how my plans to get pregnant with our second child would affect my career trajectory. But I realized, even in the months before the pandemic, that being transparent with my managers wouldn't cloud their opinion of me. They were incredibly supportive and compassionate, and I actually think it reinforced their view of me as determined.

It took a huge load off to not have to pretend with the people with whom I spent the majority of my waking hours. I didn't let everyone in, and I didn't always wear my heart on my sleeve, but the freedom to be vulnerable when I wanted was a gift. Not everyone is so lucky. I spoke with patients who suffered in silence at work, navigating losses and appointments and injections without telling a soul, fearing that being open about their fertility issues would taint their reputations, affect their careers. "I report to people who don't give two shits that I'm going through fertility treatment," one woman who works a high-powered, demanding corporate job told me.

There were times I felt innately compelled to be open with the people close to me, to bring them into my dark and swirling mind. There were times, though, when I wanted to cocoon. During the pandemic, with our social life reduced to nearly nothing, I could quite easily hide. When I was craving a distraction or support, I would emerge for long walks with one of my dearest friends, the forward ambulation and fresh air at once calming and invigorating. She knew me well enough to know that I didn't want false reassurances; I wanted to vent my grievances—with my body, with my doctors, with fate.

On April 29, 2020, the Canadian Fertility and Andrology Society released a statement recognizing that public-health officials were starting to see a "flattening of the curve"—that is, the country was seeing more recovered than active cases. Clinics, the society said, needed to prepare for a gradual and safe resumption of services. That same day, we received an email from Hannam stating that the clinic would be resuming in-person treatment in phases, beginning the following month. On June 3, 2020, our nurse emailed to let us know that the clinic was ready to resume embryo transfers. "Omg YAY!!!!!!" I responded. "I'm seeing signs of my period today, so was going to email you later today or tmrw when it fully starts. But I will call it into the nursing line:) Best news."

My transfer plan was already in place, outlining the medications I would take to prime my body to welcome an embryo. Most doctors say that before an embryo is transferred, the uterine lining should be about seven or eight millimetres thick, with a trilaminar (triple line) pattern associated with receptivity. My transfer protocol involved applying estrogen patches to my stomach and taking low dose aspirin, which is believed to increase blood flow to the uterus. "Continue until endometrial lining is ready (ideally triple line pattern and equal to or greater than 8.0 mm)," my plan said.

Once the lining was determined to be in good shape, I would add in two other medications: Prometrium, which is progesterone in tablet form that I would insert vaginally, and progesterone in oil, which I would inject into my upper tush. Progesterone is responsible for preparing the uterine lining to be receptive to implantation, and it also stimulates glands in the lining to secrete nutrients to support the development of the embryo. On the sixth day of progesterone, the transfer would take place.

On the morning of June 8, 2020, I went into the clinic for bloodwork and an ultrasound to begin my transfer cycle. Later that day, I stuck four estrogen patches to my stomach, feeling hopeful as I applied the clear adhesives. I would need to change them every two days, all the peeling and reapplying leaving behind a patchwork of red rectangles and sticky goo on my bloated tummy. If you know, you know. After just over two weeks on the patches, I headed to the clinic for my lining check. Given that I'd just recently had surgery to remove the scar tissue in my uterus, we were hopeful my lining was rejuvenated and I'd pass the test.

I didn't. An ultrasound showed that despite the surgery and the estrogen supplementation, my lining measured four millimetres and didn't have the triple-line pattern. A thin lining can result from several factors, including estrogen deficiency, chronic infection of the endometrial cells and uterine fibroids. In my case, it was safe to assume that it was due to the adhesions from the D&C. I didn't know this at the time, but Asherman's syndrome is among the most intractable causes of a thin lining. It's possible to get and stay pregnant with a thin lining that lacks the coveted triple-line pattern, but it's less likely.

On a phone call the day after our lining check, Dr. Hannam explained that a thin endometrium can be difficult to overcome, but there were some steps we could take that may help. This could have been the moment we realized I might not be able to carry a pregnancy because my uterus might not support implantation, but it wasn't. Instead, all we heard was all the ways we could fix me.

I can't remember if we asked about acupuncture or if someone at Hannam mentioned it to us, but I recall Dr. Hannam saying something along the lines of *There isn't good evidence to support that acupuncture makes a difference for a thin lining, but I don't see the harm in it and some patients find it relaxing and want to know they're doing anything and everything they can.* I was one of those patients. I asked to be connected with a team of acupuncturists who specialize in reproductive health and see their clients in Hannam's procedures area. I also started taking supplements such as L-arginine and vitamin E, which are thought to increase blood flow to the uterus.

In addition, Dr. Hannam told us about a new and unpublished uterine dilation technique he had performed on a handful of patients with a thin lining, several of whom went on to carry. The thinking is that by dilating the uterus and causing the walls to expand, any scar tissue or tighter areas would be loosened, allowing for fresh bloodflow and increased activity in the endometrial receptors.

When your goal is a baby, you'll do anything, pay what your means allow. You need to feel like you did everything, tried everything. What's worse than something not working? Not doing it and wondering if it would have, feeling like you wasted a cycle not trying it. So I scheduled the $500 uterine dilation procedure. I booked twice-weekly acupuncture appointments at $150 per visit. I was on board with including vaginal Viagra in my next transfer protocol, in the hopes that it would increase blood flow to my uterine lining. Doctors and research left me with the impression that these measures could potentially help and likely wouldn't hurt.

Seems I got the wrong impression. I later learned that a clinical practice guideline from the Canadian Fertility and Andrology Society says "there is minimal evidence to support any specific protocols or adjuvants to significantly improve pregnancy outcomes in patients with thin endometrium." Nonetheless, throwing spaghetti at the wall gave me a sense that maybe I had some modicum of power over what happened next. It was a feeling I hadn't felt in a while. Control, after all, is one of the most tragic casualties in the exercise of baby-making. At some point, usually pretty early on, you realize you're at the mercy of your body and you're pushing up against the limits of what modern science can do for you.

You're just a patient at a clinic, waiting your turn.

First, Do No Harm

IN THE SPRING of 1995, the *Orange County Register* broke a story that would earn the newspaper a Pulitzer Prize. Journalists Susan Kelleher and Kim Christensen reported that the head of the University of California Irvine Center for Reproductive Health took eggs from a woman without her consent and gave them to another patient, who went on to deliver a baby boy.

"If those allegations hold up, they would be the most serious violation of ethical trust that I am aware of in the field of reproductive technology," Dr. Arthur Caplan, then director of biomedical ethics at the University of Pennsylvania, told the paper at the time. "There may be worse things that one could do in operating a fertility clinic, but I don't know what they are."

By the fall of 1995, the *Register* reported that at least sixty women were unknowingly involved in illicit egg or embryo transfers by doctors at the UCI facility, making the case one of the biggest medical scandals in American history. It garnered international headlines and prompted a series of probes, including by the FBI and the state senate. The doctors at the centre of the scandal fled to Mexico and

Chile. The case, which led to dozens of court settlements worth tens of millions of dollars, took years to unravel.

"I have children, and I don't know where they're at," one of the affected patients told the *Los Angeles Times* in 2006. According to the *Times*, the patient learned in 2002 that her eggs and embryos had been stolen and implanted into another woman, who gave birth to twins. "I feel so cheated and so betrayed," she said.

The saga reached into Canada, affecting patients who had travelled to the UCI clinic for fertility treatment. Among them was Dr. Arthur Leader and his wife. In a phone call decades later, Dr. Leader, a reproductive endocrinologist himself, told me that during his wife's first stimulation cycle at the clinic in advance of a planned egg retrieval, she had grown somewhere in the order of sixty follicles. That's a big number. So big, in fact, that it put his wife at a high risk for severe ovarian hyperstimulation syndrome, which Dr. Leader knew could have implications for her reproductive health. The doctors were keen to move forward with the procedure, but Dr. Leader intervened and cancelled the retrieval. On the next cycle, the doctors pursued a milder stimulation protocol. The retrieval and subsequent transfer of a fresh embryo went ahead as planned, but unfortunately it didn't take. Dr. Leader and his wife had been told they had no surplus embryos, so they went ahead and did another retrieval, this time in Europe at a clinic that specialized in ICSI. That transfer was successful, and they welcomed a baby girl.

A couple of years later, Dr. Leader and his wife received an alarming letter from the Superior Court of California. It said that the couple had in fact created five other embryos, which doctors at the clinic had surreptitiously cryopreserved without their knowledge or consent. Dr. Leader said the additional embryos hadn't been transferred into other women, but the news was, of course, deeply upsetting. Dr. Leader and his wife had gone to California for treatment because he had a professional relationship with the doctors who headed the UCI clinic. "I trusted them," he said. "It was a betrayal on so many levels." Dr. Leader and his wife received another letter stating that their newly discovered embryos had been transferred to the California Cryobank for storage. In the end, they decided to dispose of the embryos because they had no confidence that they had been made from their own eggs and sperm. "What happened to us is part of the reason I'm so passionate about oversight in fertility," he said.

The University of California case is a worst-case scenario. Although this sort of situation is extremely rare, cases of this nature are not unheard of. There have been mix-ups of embryos that have resulted in women having to relinquish custody of the child they carried. In one case in the United States, two women who unknowingly grew each other's embryos ended up exchanging babies upon learning of the mix-up a few months after delivering.

In a high-profile case in Canada, Ontario fertility doctor Norman Barwin inseminated many women with the wrong sperm and, in some cases, his own. In 2016, a woman named Rebecca Dixon learned that her mother had not been inseminated with her father's sperm but rather with Dr. Barwin's. Court documents say she discovered that she is a genetic match with Dr. Barwin and various other half siblings who were conceived the same way. A class-action lawsuit was certified and grew to include approximately 250 people, including at least seventeen who learned they were conceived using Dr. Barwin's sperm and more than eighty who were conceived using donor sperm not from the chosen donor.

"How can the damages suffered by a child who discovers such a situation be measured?" an Ontario Superior Court justice wrote in approving a $13.375-million settlement in 2021. "After all, had there been a different genetic origin, that particular child would not have existed." Under the terms of the settlement, patients and their children were entitled to as much as $50,000 each in compensation, depending on their situation. Dr. Barwin, who has admitted no wrongdoing, was not personally responsible for paying out the settlement; the damages were covered by a professional medical association.

Health Canada inspection records dating back to the late 1990s suggest Dr. Barwin's clinic had on a number of occasions violated federal regulations, regarding handling of sperm, record-keeping, patient consents and more. The documents include communication between Health Canada and the Ottawa clinic, apparently attempting to work through the violations. Despite the inspectors' concerns, the clinic was deemed compliant. It didn't fail an inspection until 2010. In a document from that year, government officials wrote that while sperm regulations were aimed at preventing the transmission of infectious disease to recipients of donor sperm, the requirements were "not intended to prevent mix-up incidents."

In 2012, Dr. Barwin voluntarily stopped offering insemination services while the College of Physicians and Surgeons of Ontario investigated complaints against him. The college revoked his medical licence in 2019 after a disciplinary panel found he had impregnated women with the wrong sperm. "Your behaviour has been beyond reprehensible," the panel wrote in a public rebuke. "Your patients represent a group who were vulnerable and who placed themselves and their families completely in your trust. You betrayed that trust and by your actions deeply affected individuals and their families and cause irreparable damage that will span generations." Dr. Barwin pleaded no contest to the allegations. Through his lawyer, Dr. Barwin declined my request for comment.

There are other, less dramatic examples of human error in fertility treatment. Again, these are infrequent, but they do happen. One woman I spoke with said her clinic "forgot" to biopsy her embryos before freezing them, so she was unable to get them genetically tested. She went on to have a miscarriage after her first transfer. To this day, she wonders if that could have been avoided had her embryos been tested. This same woman underwent a D&C to remove retained products of conception from the miscarriage—at the hands of a gynecologist who later had his medical licence suspended following a regulatory hearing due to "repeated misconduct" after ten patients complained about him to the College of Physicians and Surgeons of Ontario. (Among the complaints were allegations of making inappropriate comments and dismissing patients' concerns.) To add insult to injury, when she sought to have her untested embryos moved to another clinic to continue her treatment elsewhere, there was a period of several hours where no one could tell her where her embryos were—not the original clinic, not the transport company, not the receiving clinic.

Beyond human error and professional misconduct, there's also the potential for problems when it comes to the medications and devices themselves. There have been lawsuits and settlements pertaining to defective cryopreservation products, malfunctioning storage tanks, labelling errors, ineffective pharmaceuticals and other issues. Such cases have raised interesting questions in the law, including whether human reproductive material can or should constitute "property" that gives rise to corresponding legal rights. In 2015, for example, the British Columbia Court of Appeal decided that although the sale of sperm is prohibited under the law, the plaintiffs in a case involving a freezer malfunction had nonetheless produced, owned and controlled the genetic material, thus rendering it property. The university that operated the lab was liable for the damaged sperm under a statute governing property in the custody of warehouses.

As the fertility-services market becomes increasingly consolidated, a single problem at a single company can have massive ripple effects. Take, for example, Connecticut-based medical company CooperSurgical. After an increase in complaints regarding three associated lots of its liquid embryo culture, the company recalled some of its products. "Performance issues may lead to impaired embryo development prior to the blastocyst stage," the U.S. Food and Drug Administration said in its 2024 notice, citing the manufacturer's reason for the recall. The number of affected patients is estimated to be in the thousands. (CooperSurgical didn't respond to my requests for comment.)

Among them are Jasmin and Andrew, the Vancouver Island couple who received financial assistance from the Modern Miracle Foundation to help pay for their second retrieval, which was allegedly affected by the faulty embryo culture. Their three precious embryos stopped growing sometime between day three and day six post-retrieval. Not a single one survived. "You trust that everything is working as it should," Jasmin said. "Especially if you're spending all this money." It was—and still is—deeply upsetting for them to think about the possibility that one of those embryos could have been their first baby. Andrew, who was suspicious from the outset of the fertility industry and of the incentive structures at play, became increasingly concerned that he and Jasmin were being taken for a ride. The couple found it difficult to trust their doctors, to trust the technology, to trust the process. "We never anticipated or thought of this," Jasmin said.

For Dr. Leader, who has retired from clinical practice, the Barwin case exposed several gaps in the Canadian regulatory landscape. He is among those calling on lawmakers to conduct a parliamentary review of the federal laws governing assisted human reproduction. He's deeply concerned about all the ways patients are vulnerable to being taken advantage of in an industry that's increasingly privatized.

It has been more than two decades since Canada passed its first piece of legislation governing the area of fertility care, known as the 2004 Assisted Human Reproduction Act. Although laws and regulations aren't necessarily sexy or riveting, in the context of fertility, I have found them fascinating for their intersection with ethics, morality, science and questions about the future of our species. Entire books have been dedicated to the subject of fertility law. I have sought here to be concise in relaying what I believe to be the highlights, based on conversations with lawyers, doctors and academics who have spent their careers thinking about these big issues.

The stated aim of Canada's Assisted Human Reproduction Act is to protect those who use or who are born of assisted reproductive technologies. The act prohibits, for example, creating a human clone or maintaining an embryo outside the body beyond the fourteenth day of development. The act included the creation of a federal agency to oversee the implementation of the act and the development of regulations. In 2010, though, the country's Supreme Court struck down parts of the legislation as unconstitutional, saying it infringed on provincial and territorial jurisdiction. In the end, the oversight agency was dissolved, and the responsibility to administer and enforce what remained of the act fell to Health Canada.

The legislation is quite narrowly focused on regulating donor eggs and sperm, as well as the reimbursement of expenses incurred by donors and surrogates. Over the years, the federal government has strengthened parts of the law, but critics say some aspects are outdated, lack teeth and are not enforced in any meaningful way. Canadian fertility lawyer Kelly Jordan told me she believes the act is "far too blunt an instrument to deal with the complexities of family building . . . It's an empty piece of legislation that criminalizes certain things and doesn't really regulate much of anything."

Part of the problem, experts say, is the patchwork of oversight across the country. Health Canada is responsible for enforcing rules related to how donor sperm and eggs are processed before they get distributed, imported or used in Canada. Facilities that process sperm and eggs are required, for example, to screen donors for potential infectious diseases that could impact the recipient or the child born through assisted reproduction. Health Canada has an online registry of its inspection findings, which include the reasons a clinic may be deemed non-compliant.

Beyond that, the matter of how and by whom a fertility clinic is regulated depends very much on where the facility is located and, to some degree, whether it offers publicly funded cycles. It also depends on what exactly the clinic offers. In Ontario, for example, clinics that offer "twilight" sedation are regulated under a provincial inspection program that covers facilities performing procedures outside a hospital using different levels of anesthesia.

I spoke with a nurse who has extensive experience doing inspections and creating policies. She is now a compliance expert who helps providers ensure they're operating in accordance with their jurisdiction's applicable regulatory programs. She described looking at a clinic's logbook where the ultrasound technician is supposed to record the times at which they put a probe into a disinfecting solution and then removed it. These are the probes that go into patients' vaginas. "The staff member was prefilling out the logbook before actually doing the work," she said. "You may have superb policies and procedures," she said, "but if no one is following them, that's a problem."

Dr. Leader said that because the provinces, territories, federal government and professional colleges all have authority over some aspect of fertility treatment in Canada, the buck stops with everyone and no one. "Right now in Canada, it's a free-for-all," Dr. Leader said. "A patient doesn't know, for their particular problem, for example, what a clinic's success rate is. The consumer doesn't really know what they're buying."

Clinics in Canada aren't mandated to publicly disclose their success rates, and most clinic staff, outside of nurses and doctors, aren't required to report errors. How then are patients supposed to know which one to choose? This is classically Canadian. As a journalist, I have on many occasions confronted reporting roadblocks due to data either not being collected or not being made public. Reporters here often have to file access-to-information requests with public bodies to get data that is readily available in countries like the United States.

Under the Fertility Clinic Success Rate and Certification Act, American clinics are required to report data on the fertility cycles started and carried out in their facilities, along with the outcomes, for each calendar year. The result is a searchable map of the country, published on the Centers for Disease Control and Prevention website, that provides data on factors such as the ages of patients and their reasons for using assisted reproductive technologies and on outcomes such as the percentage of embryo transfers that resulted in live births.

Although Ontario clinics are obligated to provide data on publicly funded cycles to a provincial registry, the figures are published in aggregate. Providing data on privately funded cycles in Ontario is not mandatory. Even if some clinics opted to publish their success rates voluntarily, there is no standardized system so it would be tough to make illuminating comparisons between providers. And although most Canadian IVF centres voluntarily report their data to the country's national registry, the information, again, is published in aggregate.

There are arguments against disclosure. The primary one is that it could affect a clinic's decision to take on a patient. If a patient presents with a particularly challenging case, the clinic may choose to pass on it to avoid negatively impacting its success rates. How real is this concern? Does the possible impact on inclusivity and access trump the desire for transparency? One could argue that the United States has found a way around these concerns, in part by publishing a detailed breakdown of success rates by age category and by patient versus donor eggs. That way, people can look at the data most relevant to their own situations and make their own inferences.

Because Canadian clinics don't have to report their success rates, they can, at least theoretically, do relatively poorly statistically speaking and still have a relatively successful business. Several doctors told me that the incentive structure in Canada is such that better outcomes don't necessarily mean more revenues. In fact, the opposite can be true. The more retrievals or transfers it takes to reach a pregnancy, the more the clinic can make on a per patient basis. A clinic could do well financially by offering low-quality, low-cost services at a high volume.

"In medicine, you take an oath; there's a fairly stringent screening process in selecting medical students and all that," said Dr. Taerk, the Toronto reproductive endocrinologist. "You hope that physicians are practising in good faith. Listen, it's a business. Are there physicians who are pushing patients through multiple cycles? Sure. But to have patients miserable and going through multiple cycles with a poor prognosis is a burden on all aspects of the clinic, including nurses. The more honest, transparent, on-the-level and non-revenue-generating focus you have, the better your reputation will be and the better your clinic will do . . . If patients trust you, then whatever your recommendation is won't be viewed as having ulterior motives."

In conversations with fertility patients, I confirmed that something that was true for Dan and me held true for many others: As time goes on and as the bad news rolls in, your standard of proof that something could help you get or stay pregnant becomes foolishly low. You would eat gravel if someone told you it may help. You hang onto any small tweak to your protocol as the potential difference maker. You lose your scruples along the way. You get sucked into woo-woo "medicine." Not only that, you become suspicious that your clinic sees you more as a source of income than as a person. Surely, most doctors in the reproductive health-care space are ethical and good, practising safe, scientifically supported medicine in the hopes of making their patients' dreams come true. But the structure of fertility care creates the potential for patients to be taken advantage of. And even if they're not being taken for a ride, they're likely to feel that way at some point.

One obvious way this plays out is in the rising use of treatment add-ons, which are the optional, non-essential tests and interventions that patients might be offered and billed for; these treatments may not be supported by evidence or may cause unnecessary harm. Add-ons include pre-implantation genetic testing for chromosome abnormalities, immunological treatments to reduce natural killer cell activity in cases of recurrent miscarriage or repeated implantation failure, and endometrial receptivity analysis to try to pinpoint the ideal time to transfer an embryo. These add-ons cost anywhere from a couple hundred to a few thousand dollars each.

Supporters of IVF add-ons argue that providing patients with the option of interventions that are unproven but make good biological sense has the effect of improving patient autonomy. Opponents note that beyond the added cost and the creation of false hope, doctors have a responsibility to only offer effective, evidence-based treatments that are unlikely to cause harm.

"As a consumer, you're not told that most of the add-ons that are being offered are useless," Dr. Leader said. "Where the clinics make their money is on the add-ons, just like a car dealership." National data, he said, shows a continuing upward trend in Canada for add-ons, including ICSI, assisted hatching, genetic testing and endometrial receptor analysis. The Canadian data registry, for instance, shows that the percent of frozen embryo transfers with pre-implantation genetic testing for aneuploidy climbed from 21 percent in 2019 to nearly 38 percent in 2024. Our IVF journey included several add-ons, for a total additional cost over numerous treatment rounds of $25,000.

Nowhere did I feel more like a guinea pig grasping at straws than when I was lying in a dimly lit room with electro-acupuncture needles in my stomach, legs and feet, hoping the stimulation of the fascia and muscles would cause my uterine lining to become fluffy and receptive. One time, the acupuncturist turned up the frequency on the cables connected to the needles sticking out of my lower body. A shock shot through my left foot, which involuntarily swung upward and nearly struck the acupuncturist in the face.

What the hell was I doing.

When we think about add-ons and unproven technologies in fertility treatment, it's natural for the mind to wander to the future and how artificial intelligence could improve or even transform how we make and grow babies. Researchers and tech companies around the world are exploring how science and AI can be leveraged in the fertility space, from embryo development and selection to patient communication and semen analysis.

Perhaps the most sci-fi example of an emerging technology is the artificial womb. Artificial womb technologies are experimental medical devices that mimic the uterine environment. Even a couple of weeks of gestation can make the difference between life and death in a premature baby. Research teams have had some success using artificial wombs to gestate premature lamb and pig fetuses ex utero. One of the devices, called a biobag, features synthetic amniotic fluid, catheters that imitate an umbilical cord and an oxygenator that ensures sufficient oxygen delivery.

Artificial womb technology raises the question: If you can grow a preterm baby outside the human body, could there come a time when artificial wombs replace uteruses entirely? Might there be a day when people no longer have to get pregnant in order for the human species to reproduce and survive? If I had been living in the year, say, 2050 instead of 2020, would the state of my uterus have been immaterial, irrelevant? It's hard to know what the future holds, of course, and there are limits to what science can achieve. What works for a lamb or a pig might not work for a human.

Artificial wombs for humans might be a thing of the future, but there are already examples of far less ethically charged AI applications and technological advances in the fertility space. While some doctors and clinics are entrenched in their ways, with no obvious interest in evolving, others are embracing the new frontier. Some are hiring staff dedicated specifically to figuring out how AI could improve fertility treatment and the patient experience.

"The future is automated," Dr. Daneshmand said. "When things are automated, you have much less deviation from what's supposed to happen." He pointed to the growing use of robots that digitally identify, track, monitor and store frozen eggs and embryos. Advancements in embryo grading are also in the offing. Some day in the not-so-distant future, Dr. Daneshmand said, AI machines will be relied on to rank embryos based on thousands of images in a database.

Dr. Dan Nayot, a Toronto-based reproductive endocrinologist and medical director of The Fertility Partners, spoke about myriad AI advances at the Canadian Fertility and Andrology Society conference I attended in September 2023, including an AI application that automatically identifies, counts and measures ovarian follicles in a matter of seconds via transvaginal ultrasound and predicts the optimal timing for an egg retrieval; a technology that evaluates endometrial receptivity and uses a scoring system based on what research predicts will be the quality of the lining at the time of an embryo transfer; and an AI application that predicts which eggs are likelier to develop into blastocysts.

"I think of AI as a baseball game," said Dr. Nayot, who is also a co-founder of Future Fertility, a med-tech start-up that applies AI in the field of assisted reproductive medicine. "I think we're maybe in the bottom of the second, top of the third . . . There are going to be issues and hiccups, but I do believe it's here to stay."

Breaking

"I HAVE TO tell you something," my sister said over the phone. "I'm so nervous. I feel so bad."

Alone in our bedroom at the family cottage outside Toronto, I sank to the floor. I knew what was coming. "It's okay," I said.

"I'm pregnant," Mackenzie said through tears. "I don't know why I'm crying. I'm sorry. I just feel so bad. I was so nervous to tell you. It's early. I just took a test a couple of days ago."

"It's okay," I repeated. "I'm happy for you. I know you guys wanted this. It's okay."

A jumble of thoughts raced through my mind. I could tell she was confident she would actually have this baby, that she wouldn't miscarry it, as I had three times. I marvelled at how sure she sounded. I felt jealous she felt free to be sure. Her son had just turned one in March, and this baby was coming in February, so she would have two under two. I felt her pity, and I despised it. I hated knowing that someone felt sorry for me, like I was some kind of wounded bird that people tiptoed around. I felt sick that this was the dynamic between us. I was happy for her. Genuinely. This girl is the kindest person I know, and I want nothing but a full and easy life for her. But I was sad for me. I was so very sad for me.

The spring and summer of 2020 can only be described as a hellscape of hormones and cancelled transfer cycles. Despite the uterine lining dilation procedure, the estrogen patches and suppositories, the vaginal Viagra, the supplements and the acupuncture sessions, my lining wouldn't get past four millimetres and it never achieved triple-line status. We had genetically balanced embryos waiting for us, frozen in time. They were ready to grow with nowhere to go. We were at an impasse.

Around the time Mackenzie called with her news, Dr. Hannam recommended that we take a two-month break from treatment to let my endometrial receptors rejuvenate. Sometimes, he said, your body just needs a break. We resisted the idea of a break at first. We couldn't fathom "wasting time doing nothing," waiting helplessly as Sid, now two and a half, continued to grow up without a brother or sister. But I knew deep down that I needed a break. I needed to be free.

There's so much you can't or shouldn't do when you're in the throes of IVF and all the hormones and procedures it involves. Make solid plans, feel like yourself, comfortably wear pants, wake up feeling rested, go swimming, exercise so hard your face turns tomato red, drink alcohol, have a bath. I was sick of it. I was sick of the appointments, the needles, the red marks on my bloated stomach. I was sick of the probes up my vagina and the green discharge coming out of it from the Viagra suppositories. I was sick of my hair falling out from all the hormonal ups and downs. I was sick of getting phone calls from the clinic and hearing our nurse say "I'm sorry, but . . ." I was sick of bad news always lurking around the corner. I was sick of taking dozens of pills every day, feeling nauseous from them. I was sick of not having sex when I wanted to. The toll of IVF on a couple's sex life is real. Sex loses its magic and becomes something you have to manage, something you try not to resent. I was sick of not living my life. I was sick of not feeling like me. I was sick of not *being* me.

One former IVF patient put it to me this way: "I was gluten-free, alcohol-free, dairy-free, fun-free for all the years I was trying to grow my family. When I was done, I was like, 'Let me abuse my body after making it a temple.'"

I relished in the reclamation of my body. For the first time in a long time, I wasn't on hormones, coming off hormones, or about to start hormones. I drank as much coffee as I wanted, had a glass of wine when I felt like it, went for runs and bike rides, had baths, jumped in the lake, made plans and kept them. For those two months, I felt like I could breathe again. The name *Hannam* wasn't about to light up on my phone with results or medication instructions. I felt temporarily released from the shackles of IVF.

And I read. I devoured Glennon Doyle's memoir *Untamed*. The themes—about striving and being good, about living in a state of "should," about making peace with our bodies—resonated deeply. One particular passage took my breath away. It challenged me to meet my fears with curiosity, to trust that pain gives way to a rising. The distinction between pain and suffering had never occurred to me. I had thought of the two as inextricable. But I was wrong. Pain is unavoidable. Suffering is not.

Looking back on this time, when I was undeniably suffering, I don't think I was a very good friend to those who were used to having me at their side. It's the ugly truth. Call it selfish or an act of self-preservation, I pulled back from loved ones who were pregnant or who had just had their second babies. One of those people was my close friend. She had a baby one month after the pandemic was declared. It was a terrifying time to be pregnant, to deliver, to have a newborn. I wasn't there for her. Not because I didn't want to be. But because I didn't know how to be. I didn't know how to support a friend who was in a situation I would have given my right arm to be in.

I also withdrew from social media. I couldn't see one more pregnancy or birth announcement, one more bump pic or black-and-white photo of a tiny baby nestled on a woman's chest, a tired smile on her face, eyes filled with tears. I turned inward. When you're going through infertility, your world often becomes smaller, like a camera lens narrowing and narrowing until it's a pinhole.

At the same time, I became closer with friends in fertility struggles themselves. One of them had just watched his wife suffer a miscarriage after multiple rounds of IVF. We commiserated in our shared plight. We offered each other words of support. I sent him the Glennon Doyle pain passage. He sent me a quote from his friend who is a fertility doctor: "Those who have the fortitude to continue with the process eventually tend to make magic."

If I said that I didn't think about what my lining was doing inside me over the course of that two-month break, I would be lying. I wanted to carry our second child, but we were realizing that we needed to start getting comfortable with the idea that I might not. "As part of your story, I think it is reasonable to look into surrogacy," Dr. Hannam wrote in a July 28, 2020, clinical note. He stated there was, at best, a 20 percent chance for implantation in a uterus that looked like mine. He added that even if a transfer was successful, I would be at a higher risk for pregnancy complications such as placenta accreta, in which the placenta embeds into the uterine wall and can cause life-threatening hemorrhaging when it detaches.

People sometimes ask me if we considered adoption at this juncture. The answer is sort of, not really. The time to think about that might have been after the third miscarriage, before we started fertility treatment. It had felt premature then, and it felt too late now. I'd already done two retrievals. Our future babies were on ice, and we just needed a safe place for them to grow. We were all in on IVF.

This might sound strange or unexpected, but I wasn't particularly emotional about the prospect of turning to surrogacy at this stage in our quest. I think that's largely because I was still hopeful—pretty convinced, even—that I would end up carrying. We were still trying to get *me* pregnant, so I was in a good headspace to start exploring what it would look like to get someone else pregnant. It felt prudent, and hopefully unnecessary, to do some research online and talk to people who had had babies via surrogacy.

I learned that there are two kinds of surrogacy: traditional, in which the carrier provides the egg and is therefore genetically linked to the child (it dates back to the Book of Genesis, in which Abraham impregnated his servant, Hagar, so that he and his wife, Sarah, could have a child); and gestational, in which the egg and sperm that form an embryo come from the intended parents or from third-party donors or both. In this version of surrogacy, the embryo is then transferred into the uterus of the surrogate, who has no genetic connection to the resulting child.

Gestational surrogacy is today the most common form of surrogacy. And it's becoming increasingly prevalent. That being said, it's still quite rare in the scheme of things; in 2024 in Canada, surrogates were involved in 1,306 embryo transfers, or 4.7 percent of total transfers. The model in Canada is one of altruistic surrogacy, in which a person is expected to carry a pregnancy to term out of the goodness of her heart. It's illegal to compensate a person to act as a surrogate, and it's illegal to make or accept payment to arrange for the services of a surrogate. It's also against the law to pay a donor for their sperm or eggs. Any of those criminal offences could result in a fine of up to $500,000, imprisonment for up to ten years or both.

Although people in Canada can't compensate surrogates in the country, they can reimburse them for reasonable expenses and lost work-related income during pregnancy. Most people don't personally know someone willing and able to get pregnant for them. So how are people like Dan and me supposed to find a surrogate? There are two main avenues: through an agency or through an independent search, which usually involves social media. A third approach, augmenting an independent search with the support of a marketing consultant, is increasing in popularity.

Agencies use various channels to build their roster, reaching potential gestational carriers through social media and word of mouth. Wait times to match with a surrogate vary by agency, but intended parents are typically quoted somewhere between six and twelve months. It can be shorter or longer. One thing is clear though: There are far more intended parents than there are surrogates.

Who are these women? And since surrogates can't be compensated, why would anyone want to do it? It's a good question, and it's one that a group of researchers in Canada went to great lengths to try to answer. As part of the Surrogates' Voices project, researchers administered a survey in 2022 to people who had been surrogates in Canada since 2004; 174 surrogates responded. The surrogates could choose more than one reason for carrying someone else's child and responded like so: 86 percent said they wanted to help others, 62 percent said they specifically wanted to help strangers become parents, 49 percent said they enjoyed being pregnant, and 12 percent reported wanting the "financial benefits" of surrogacy. "Surrogates are more likely to be white, very slightly less well-educated, Canadian citizens, and more likely to be married or in a common-law relationship, when compared with women of a similar age," said Professor Alana Cattapan, one of the project's researchers and the Canada Research Chair in the Politics of Reproduction at the University of Waterloo. "It doesn't tend to be people who belong to marginalized communities or are low income."

The founder and owner of one of Canada's largest surrogacy agencies, Canadian Fertility Consulting (CFC), said many surrogates sign up with the agency out of a desire to be part of a community. The motive, Leia Swanberg said, should be more than a desire to carry a baby for someone else, because there's no guarantee that they will have a successful journey. And while money isn't a key motivator, the surrogate may enjoy some "perks." "It could be the difference between Heinz ketchup and No Name ketchup," Ms. Swanberg said, referring to the reimbursement of grocery expenses a surrogate receives. "It could mean exposure to self-care—naturopathic medicines, yoga or a gym membership." She said the average age of first-time surrogates at the agency in 2024 was twenty-seven, and the median family income was between $58,000 and $75,000. The majority of the agency's surrogates, she said, live in rural areas.

In the twenty years she has been immersed in the surrogacy world, first as a surrogate herself (twice over) and later as the head of the agency, Swanberg has witnessed some shifts. With the overturning of Roe v. Wade in 2022, Americans who would have undergone surrogacy in certain parts of the United States have been looking to surrogates in Canada because they want access to abortion care should certain circumstances arise. In fact, some agencies in the United States won't match intended parents with surrogates in particular states amid fears that a surrogate would be denied an abortion even in a life-threatening emergency.

And while intended parents used to take a doctor's word for it when they gave a surrogate their stamp of approval, Swanberg said these days they're much more particular. They're more easily put off by a surrogate's use of an antidepressant or ADHD medication or by their BMI. With the rise of wellness culture and weight-loss drugs, she said, the agency has been seeing a lot of "fatphobia." Intended parents are also squeamish about the recreational use of cannabis, which is legalized in Canada and parts of the United States. "The thinking is 'I don't want a stoner carrying my kid,'" she said. "Well, it's legalized and if [the surrogate] says she's not going to use it during pregnancy, then what's the problem?"

The demand for surrogacy comes from within Canada but also from abroad. The Surrogates' Voices research found that somewhere in the order of 50 percent of Canadian surrogates carry for international intended parents. This is in part because Canada is economically attractive, due to the altruistic surrogacy model and the existence of high-quality universal health care. The main reason the country attracts international intended parents, though, is simple and unrelated to money: Surrogacy in Canada is legal.

I was surprised to learn surrogacy is outlawed or extremely limited in many countries, including throughout much of Europe. Intended parents in countries such as France, Spain and Germany look to surrogacy-friendly jurisdictions like Canada and parts of the United States for help building their families. The demand has driven up the costs associated with surrogacy, and wait times. (Some U.S. states limit surrogacy to intended parents who are heterosexual residents using their own gametes, while others don't recognize surrogacy contracts and consider them to be void and unenforceable.) Italy has taken an especially hard line against surrogacy, in the name of protecting women. Not only is it prohibited in the country, lawmakers also passed legislation in 2024 making it illegal for intended parents in Italy to pursue surrogacy abroad. The law makes it a punishable offence—with steep fines or imprisonment—to impregnate a surrogate abroad and bring the baby home.

Because there are far more intended parents than there are surrogates in Canada, surrogates can be selective when it comes to deciding who they want to work with. Do they want to do a journey with someone married or single? Gay or straight? (Some surrogates prefer to work with gay men because they find it easier interacting with intended fathers than with intended mothers, who may struggle with not being the one to carry.) Someone wanting to have their first child? Religious or atheist? From within their own province or elsewhere in Canada? Abroad? Surrogates typically choose intended parents who already have several embryos banked and ready for transfer. Otherwise, they run the risk of matching with someone who has trouble creating embryos, which would prolong the process or, worse yet, end it before it really begins. Another primary consideration in the matching process relates to views on termination. Do the surrogate and intended parents share similar thoughts on terminating a pregnancy for medical or any other reasons?

If intended parents opt to go the agency route, they fill out a profile and make a short video about who they are and why they're looking for help growing a family. Surrogates then review the profile and decide whether they want to be introduced. What follows, effectively, is an exercise in matchmaking—a high-stakes dating period, which usually lasts about two weeks. When the time is up, the surrogate and intended parents decide whether they want to move forward together.

The agency is also there to guide the parties through the process, including recommending fertility lawyers, helping to negotiate the legal agreement, finding a therapist or social worker to do the psychological screening required by most fertility clinics to proceed, managing expenses, navigating the relationship, answering questions and working through challenges that may arise.

The fee structures, we learned through our consultation calls, differ by agency, but typically an intended parent pays the agency a smallish sum to sign up and get put on the waitlist and then pays a significant "consulting fee" upon matching with a surrogate. The companies we spoke with in the summer of 2020 quoted us consulting fees totalling between $12,000 and $16,000. In addition to the fees associated with finding a match, there are also fees for crafting the legal agreement, medical screening, psychological screening, obtaining life insurance for the surrogate, medications, maternity clothes, gas and mileage for going to appointments, prenatal vitamins, time off work, housekeeping, childcare support if needed and, of course, the embryo transfer itself. "Plan for $60–80k, but will likely be closer to $45–50k," I wrote down in my notes from a call with one of the agencies. The costs vary greatly depending on a number of factors, including whether, for example, the intended parents need to pay for a surrogate's lost wages and childcare costs if she has to go on bedrest.

If we moved forward with surrogacy, one agency explained to me, we would have to deposit $20,000 into a reimbursement account they would manage. This account would need to be topped up over the course of the pregnancy, to cover the surrogate's out-of-pocket expenses. The agency would send us a monthly account statement, showing the withdrawals, deposits and remaining balance. Any funds remaining in the account at the end would be returned to us. The time from match to embryo transfer, we were told, could be as little as two months.

Intended parents often choose to work with an agency because it provides a sense of comfort, rigor and security. As one intended parent put it to me, the agency felt like a "safety net." In reality, though, protection for everyone involved is primarily derived from the medical screening, the mental-health clearance and the legal contract. It's entirely possible—and much cheaper—to navigate surrogacy without an agency. This is what's called an independent journey. The surrogate and intended parents either already know each other or find each other through word of mouth, social media or online forums. They find their own fertility lawyers and counsellors to do the psychological evaluations, and they manage the expenses and reimbursements. Some intended parents embarking on an independent journey (and even some who are working with agencies) hire a marketing consultant to help them craft their "brand identity" and develop social-media content to capture the attention of potential surrogates.

One such consultant is Baden Colt. She runs Not My Tummy, a boutique marketing and communications firm that supports intended parents in finding their surrogate through social, digital and traditional media. An intended parent herself, she hired an agency to help her find a surrogate in 2021, but she ended up finding a carrier on her own. She posted a call-out video on Instagram that went viral, garnering roughly 700,000 views. In the short video set to catchy music that was trending at the time, her smiling husband is holding their dog and snapping his fingers as words pop into frame, describing the characteristics of the person they're looking for. It's a simple video, but there's something undeniably endearing and compelling about it. "Our agency was completely dumbfounded by this experience," recounted Colt, who has a background in marketing. "They said, 'We've never seen this: One intended parent has tens of surrogates reaching out to them.'" Her advice to clients, now that she's a consultant herself, boils down to this: "Don't lead with your diagnosis. Lead with what makes you great."

One of my friends, Monica, had her first baby via a surrogate she found through an agency. She decided to do an independent search for someone to carry their second. A friend of hers who is a social-media influencer put a call out to her followers on Instagram, asking if anyone could help Monica grow her family. Several women responded, but three seemed really serious about it. One of them "totally ghosted" her, Monica told me, another lived nearby (too close for comfort, she decided) and the third, Jennifer, seemed great (and turned out to be great; she carried Monica's second and third children).

I spoke with Jennifer, who has done four surrogacy journeys, three of them culminating in babies. She doesn't have any siblings herself, because her mother had to have a full hysterectomy due to a severe case of endometriosis. She also has friends who struggled with infertility. It was on her heart to help people in need. In the summer of 2023, while pregnant with Monica's third child, Jennifer attended a reunion of sorts in Ontario. It was an unlikely group, brought together by their shared connection with her: two gay men from France for whom she carried, their child, the woman who donated the eggs to make it possible, Monica, her husband and their two children, one of whom Jennifer had carried.

I went for a walk with Monica when we were at the outset of exploring surrogacy. She had been through it, and I had questions. I wanted to know what it was like having someone else grow your baby. I wondered if I could trust another person to grow our baby in their body, in their home, at their work, in their life.

I will never forget what she told me, a version of this: "When you find the right person—and you'll know when you do—you will trust her. Will you have to let go of some control? Yes. A lot of it. But you can't micromanage the pregnancy. You just have to trust that she will do for your baby what she did for her own. And you have to remember that at the end of the day, the real goal was never for you to get pregnant with your baby. It has always been for you to end up with a baby in your arms. That's your endgame. *Baby in arms.*"

On October 22, 2020, nearly one year after we started IVF, we got the green light to do our first transfer. My lining didn't look ideal in the ultrasound imaging, at just under six millimetres. But it had a faint indication of the triple-line pattern. It was enough for Dr. Hannam to agree that we go for it, given that we had several genetically tested embryos. The assessment would have been different if we'd had just one or two.

The feeling after a transfer is very strange. You may have just gotten yourself knocked up. You feel every twinge in your body as if it's a signal of something. Even though you know, intellectually, that putting an embryo into a uterus is kind of like placing a poppyseed into the sticky middle of a peanut butter sandwich, you wonder if going pee or coughing will cause the embryo to fall out. Your skin might break out, you might be nauseous, you might be tired, but you know that these pregnancy symptoms might only be side effects from all the hormones you're on.

Dan was extremely anxious after the transfer. He followed me around the house, hovering and doting. He would appear behind me in the bathroom as I was washing my face, beside me in the kitchen as I made breakfast, at the front door when I pulled into the driveway. At first it was cute. Then I felt suffocated by the pressure and the anticipation. I told him as much, in the nicest way possible. Before I spoke with him, I reminded myself that while it's inevitably harder to be the patient going through IVF than to be the partner, Dan was finding it difficult to be so physically removed.

Nothing was happening inside his body, so he became obsessed with what was happening in mine. The only window into that was through my communication. Even when I had nothing to report, he needed to know there was nothing to report. He needed to know that I wasn't cramping. That I hadn't bled. We had made it this far without much in the way of arguing, moving in lockstep with each decision. I was on anti-anxiety medication and had for years joked that he had meds coursing naturally through his veins. This was really the first time in our relationship that I saw him as human on the mental-health front. He, too, was capable of being paralyzed by anxiety and debilitating rumination. He had been patient and supportive of me through my anxious bouts. It was my turn to be there for him, without being judgmental or snippy. IVF for us was a lot of this. Taking turns.

We knew that a pregnancy likely wouldn't be detected by an at-home test until at least a week after the transfer. It was impossible for us to wait that long. On Wednesday, November 1, six days after the transfer, I peed on a stick. "Ugh I couldn't help myself and did a test," I wrote my sister. "And zero line . . . Probably good for me to have the reality check . . . Hoping it was just too early. Holy fuck I'm sick of this. Going to try to wait until Sunday for the next one. I really thought we'd get a faint line."

We tried to keep distracted over the next few days. Also impossible. As it happened, we had our friend's second daughter's first birthday on Saturday—the friend whom I would have been pregnant at the same time as had we not had the loss in early 2019. We were supposed to have had our second kids around the same time; now she was celebrating her younger daughter turning one and here I was not even pregnant yet, or at least not knowingly.

The birthday was at a park. For some reason, Sid, who was not quite three years old, was worried the helium balloons would lift off from the grass. I explained that the balloons were attached to ribbons on a little weight, so they were tethered to the ground. She wouldn't relent. She wouldn't stop worrying. I could relate. Things that seemed unlikely to happen seemed to keep happening. A little while later, Sid came running over to me, sobbing, pointing upward. One of the balloons—a light pink one—had somehow detached from the weight and floated off into the clear blue sky.

I woke up around 5:45 a.m. Sunday morning, rolled over in bed and nudged Dan to wake him. He was already stirring, as anxious as I was to take a test. I went to the bathroom, peed on a stick, put the light pink cap back on the end of it and took it with me into bed. We set a timer for three minutes, but I couldn't help myself and peeked.

Two pink lines. I was pregnant.

I shook with elation and relief, tears spilling out of my eyes. It didn't feel real. After all the pain and heartbreak and loss and uncertainty, I was pregnant. Those two pink lines were mine. They were ours.

I ran into the bathroom to pee on another test, a digital one, just to be sure. An hourglass blinked and blinked and then flashed "YES" with a positive plus sign. It had been so long since I'd been pregnant, about nineteen months to be exact. It should have felt familiar, but it felt different by virtue of the mechanism—IVF, not sex.

"My hands are shaking," I said in a video we recorded in bed at 5:57 a.m. "I didn't want to take a video of [us testing] because we get bad news all the time, but we just found out that apparently I'm pregnant. We're very excited but also terrified. I'm shaking. Fingers crossed." We went to the park later that day. It was weirdly warm for November. I remember feeling the sun on my face. I remember feeling like this time would be different, that I wouldn't miscarry. It was a genetically balanced embryo, and I was on hormones to support the pregnancy.

The pregnancy was confirmed with an hCG blood test the following day at the clinic. It was my mom's birthday. Telling her was the greatest gift. She had been such a source of support through our hard times. She had prayed for us, given me sage advice, sent her love and care from afar. I didn't see our journey through a religious lens, but she very much did—there was always a bigger plan, a reason to trust, to let go. There was something so comforting about it, even if I myself didn't believe. I went back for bloodwork a couple of days later to see if the levels had roughly doubled. Our nurse emailed us with the results. "It has gone up, but not as much as we were hoping," she wrote. "No special precautions until our next check. Please continue with your meds with no changes and come back again on Friday for repeat bloodwork at 8:10 a.m."

I don't know if it was psychosomatic, but I started cramping and felt like my breasts were less sore. I sunk to the bedroom floor, sobbing. Dan lay down beside me on the ground. He put his arm around me as we both cried at the seeming injustice of it all. We practically begged the clinic to let me come in sooner for bloodwork—Friday felt too far away, and I couldn't bear the thought of continuing with the injections if I had already lost the pregnancy. We decided to go for a walk through the nearby ravine. It was cloudy and threatening rain, but the clouds held off and we wandered for the better part of an hour. The cramps subsided. I pressed my breasts to see if they were sore and was confused by their tenderness.

Friday's bloodwork results landed in my inbox while I was in the kitchen fixing Sid a snack. The hCG level had more than doubled from Wednesday, a good rise and a good sign. I was shifted to the clinic's early pregnancy program and assigned a new nurse. Our first ultrasound was scheduled for November 23, 2020. Because of the pandemic, I would have to go to our ultrasounds alone.

When the day came, I texted Dan from the ultrasound appointment, saying I was "kinda terrified" but that I was praying and visualizing that all was okay. "I keep repeating: 'My body has done this successfully before. It's doing it again now,'" I wrote him. Ten minutes later, I texted him saying the technician had detected a yolk sac, the structure outside the embryo that provides nutrients to the developing pregnancy. "Too early for heartbeat," I wrote. "But she said everything looks good. Not to worry. I'll prob be asked to come back next week for the heartbeat and dating ultrasound . . . We got another fucking win!"

I left the next ultrasound, at around seven and a half weeks on November 30, with a sonogram image in hand. The technician had detected a heartbeat. Dan and I were starting to exhale. But then we got voicemail later that day with the full ultrasound report, saying that although they were able to find a heartbeat, it wasn't beating as fast as they would like to see at this stage. Again with the cautious optimism.

Looking back now, perhaps we should have been more alive to what was coming. The wonky hCG levels. The slower heartbeat. But we weren't. I wasn't. I was extremely nauseous and tired, able to stomach only bagels, chicken noodle soup, crackers and popsicles. We were totally blindsided by what happened next.

On December 7, I went to the clinic for another ultrasound. I should have been just over eight weeks by this point. I lay down on the table, nervous but not terrified, as the technician applied gel to the probe and confirmed my date of birth. I knew this technician from cycle monitoring. She wasn't the chattiest, but she was being uncharacteristically quiet as she performed the ultrasound.

"You can see a heartbeat, right?" I asked.

"I can't say anything, honey," she responded. "Just let me continue."

I looked up at the white ceiling. That damn clinic ceiling. I had stared up at it so many times, through all the ultrasounds during cycle monitoring for the retrievals and ahead of the transfer attempts. Through all the acupuncture sessions.

When the technician was done with the imaging, she led me to one of the offices in a hallway near the ultrasound rooms. I hadn't let myself cry, because I told myself I didn't know anything yet. Then a doctor I had never met walked into the room. I'm sure she told me her name, I'm sure she said all kinds of things, but all I heard was that there was no heartbeat. She was gentle in her delivery, and I will be forever grateful for that. She left the room, presumably to speak with our nurse.

I let myself go. "I can't," I sobbed, my head buried in my crossed arms on the desk, speaking to no one and everyone. "I can't. I can't.

I can't. I can't do this again. No. No. No. I can't." I will never forget what I said and felt in that room in that moment, crying uncontrollably, alone with the door slightly ajar. And then Dan walked in. He had been waiting in the lobby downstairs, and they made a compassionate exception to their COVID rules and let him into the clinic. I didn't even look up. I just kept repeating myself: "I can't. I can't. I can't." I felt his arms wrap around me, his tears on my neck, his chest vibrating against me as he cried.

It wasn't enough to have had a missed miscarriage. Because my blood type is negative and because I was inevitably going to start bleeding, I needed to get an injection that would prevent my body from making antibodies that could threaten future pregnancies. We would also need to go to a pharmacy to pick up the Mifegymiso combo to help pass the miscarriage. As the pharmacist explained how to take the medications, I could feel myself disassociating. It was as if I was floating outside my body and watching as the scene played out, as if it was happening to someone else. I couldn't believe he was talking to *me*.

When we got home, I crawled into bed and texted my parents, sister and close friend to let them know what had happened. And then I cried myself to sleep. When I woke up, the only thing I wanted to do was watch mindless reality TV. It's my medicine in emotional times. Dan would go for walks; I would curl up with my heating pad, some popcorn and a nonsense show. It helped me zone out, stop thinking, stop crying. One woman I spoke with said she called her sad days her "couch days" because they were spent so tuned into a show that she was tuned out from real life.

That afternoon, our nurse emailed me to say that the doctor I had seen had notified Dr. Hannam that no heartbeat had been detected. "I am unsure if [Dr. Hannam] will be able to call today," she said. "You are able to take the medication today as you were counselled by [the doctor]."

We had been in Dr. Hannam's care for over a year. In our lowest moment yet, we couldn't have a phone call with him? You might wonder what I would have wanted to hear. I felt uncomfortable starting the medication without speaking to my doctor. I had been so nauseous and tired leading up to the ultrasound that I was finding it hard to believe that there wasn't a heartbeat. It didn't feel real. I wasn't bleeding. I still *felt* pregnant, so I couldn't believe I wasn't anymore. I needed to hear my doctor say it. I needed something more than the naked transmission of medical fact from the mouths of people who didn't know the specifics of my case or the depths of our struggle.

Dan did dinnertime with Sid and got her ready for bed. I mustered the energy to get out from under the covers and give Sid a goodnight kiss, holding back tears as I buried my face into her neck. I didn't tell her anything about what was happening in my body, because I didn't want her to know that we were trying to have a baby. Mama just wasn't feeling well.

We will never know why I miscarried. The risk of miscarriage in women who conceive with their own eggs through IVF is not considered to be inherently higher than the risk of miscarriage in women who conceive spontaneously. Even embryos that have been cleared through pre-implantation genetic testing can still end up going sideways. Studies show that somewhere in the order of 10 percent of pregnancies resulting from the transfer of a euploid embryo result in a loss. In my case, though, was it a lining issue?

Around 9:30 p.m., Dr. Hannam called me. He couldn't tell us why we had lost the pregnancy, but he could tell us for sure that it was over. Around 10 a.m. the following morning, as instructed, I took the mifepristone. I was still in denial, so there was a part of me that felt that by taking the medication, I would be killing our baby. Intellectually, I knew that not to be the case, but I was physically sickened by what I was doing. The following morning, after taking Sid to get her scheduled flu shot, I put the misoprostol tablets in my mouth and braced myself for the physical expulsion. The symptoms that followed were as advertised: cramping more severe and sustained than the worst period cramps I'd ever endured, and enough bleeding and clotted tissue that I needed to change my pad every few hours. I took Percocet for the pain, Gravol for the nausea. I needed to sleep so that life could go on.

I'd had enough experience with miscarriage by now to know that there's a rhythm to it. I gave names to the stages. I knew I was already past the hardest part: the Finding Out. After the Finding Out, there's the Bleeding. It hurts and it's draining, but it passes. Then there's the Calm. This is the window in which the pain has subsided and you've started to accept what happened. And then there's the Reset. This is when you get your period for the first time after the loss, when you know the miscarriage is physically and hormonally behind you and your body has regained its hormonal footing. It means you can start trying again soon. If you're one of the lucky ones, you will eventually have a viable pregnancy and can enter the final stage, Baby in Arms. I didn't feel like I could move on from a miscarriage until I had a baby in my arms. I didn't fully put the 2017 miscarriage behind me until Sid was born. That's limiting and unfortunate. I wish I'd had the wherewithal and mental fortitude to move past the trauma of loss without needing a gain. I wish I didn't need to have a baby to wash myself of all the ones that never made it.

I was through the Finding Out. I was through the Bleeding and had moved into the Calm. The Reset was on the horizon. Please, please, let me get to Baby in Arms.

The unexpected loss of the pregnancy made me acutely aware of our mortality, of how our existence teeters on the razor's edge of life and death. Anything living could soon be dead. Things I thought were safe maybe weren't. I had been so sure that everything was fine with the pregnancy. The shock at the loss was destabilizing. It forced me to face the fact that life is fragile, even if we don't want to dwell on it or admit it. This made me tremendously anxious. I worried more than usual about everything. About Sid choking or getting hit by a car. About why Dan wasn't answering his phone. About what would happen to them if I died.

Around this time, my psychiatrist recommended I read *Man's Search for Meaning* by Viktor E. Frankl. I was hurting. I was willing to try anything. I ordered the book and brought it up to the cottage over the December holidays. It was a Baum family tradition to spend New Year's Eve up north at the lake. In the foreword, rabbi emeritus and author Harold S. Kushner underscores one of the book's most profound messages: You can't control what happens to you in life, but you can control how you feel and respond. No one and nothing can take that from you.

Eyes Wide Shut

WE WERE IN the Calm, but that didn't mean we weren't feverishly working to move forward with our IVF journey. At this stage in the process, that meant putting together a video and an "intended parent profile" for CFC, the surrogacy agency we had decided to work with. Our first attempt at making a two-minute video was a total failure. We thought it would be cute to include Sid in it, so the potential surrogates could see who they might be carrying a sibling for. But she was three years old and was being squirmy and goofy. I was coming off a miscarriage and had zero patience.

Our second attempt at the video, we were told by someone at the agency, didn't hit the mark. It was a bit flat and too focused on what we had gone through and why we were looking for a surrogate, as opposed to giving a sense of who we are and how we like to spend our time. For the third attempt, we recorded ourselves outside, just the two of us. Watching the video all these years later, I see a broken shell of a woman under the arm of a man trying to keep it together. I started the video with a clip of some candid footage of Sid from the summer prior. Standing on the front stoop on a sunny day and sporting sunglasses, a high ponytail and a big smile, Sid belted out her favourite song at the time. "Oh Mr. Sun, Sun, Mr. Golden Sun, please shine down on me," she sang.

We didn't know what we were doing. There was no guidebook on how to be a "good" intended parent or how to come across as one. We answered questions on the profile form as best we could. What kind of relationship were we hoping for during the pregnancy? Afterward? We weren't totally sure. All we knew was that we wanted the relationship to be organic and based on trust. We were open as to what that could look like.

The surrogacy agency started sending us brief descriptions of potential surrogates. Generally speaking, we were provided with the woman's name, her beliefs on termination, the type of intended parent she was interested in being matched with (gay couples, married couples, Canadians, international intended parents, people with or without children), province of residence, her age and BMI. Clinics have different guidelines and criteria for who they will and won't work with when it comes to gestational carriers.

It's typically recommended that surrogates are done having their own children before carrying for someone else. God forbid they experience a pregnancy or labour complication that compromises their ability to bear children. Our clinic relied on the Canadian Fertility and Andrology Society's guidelines for gestational carrier screening, which includes the following criteria: non-smoking and between the ages of twenty-one and forty-four; BMI ideally 18.5 to 24.9, though a BMI between 25 and 34.9 would be considered based on an overall health examination; a history of at least one previous uncomplicated term pregnancy; no more than a total of five previous deliveries or three births via Caesarean section; emotional and legal counselling completed. At Hannam, a workup for a surrogate included a sonohysterogram or diagnostic hysteroscopy, infectious disease testing and a mock cycle.

Among the truncated profiles we were sent was one from a woman named Stacey. Healthy BMI, Ontario, aged thirty-one, open to all couples, termination would need to be discussed with the intended parents. There was another woman who appealed to us, but we were told in a follow-up email that she was a recent smoker who had just quit. Dan and I weren't comfortable with that, though we appreciated the transparency.

We told our case specialist at the agency that we were interested in Stacey. The agency passed along our profile and video to her, and we waited. We thought it unlikely that we would match so quickly. It had only been about six weeks or so since we'd signed on with the agency. A few days later, though, the agency let us know that Stacey was interested in us as well. Though we were still planning to try at least one more transfer with me, we decided to begin the introduction process. We would be transparent with Stacey that we weren't quite ready to commit to surrogacy, but that it was looking likely that we would go that route.

The agency connected us with Stacey by email, kicking off a ten-day introduction period of phone calls, emails and text messages. In the Before Pandemic times, if the potential surrogate and intended parents lived in close enough proximity, they could meet in person. Some intended parents want to visit the surrogate at her home so they can see where and how she lives and get comfortable with picturing where their baby might grow. The agency was clear that if the match was a success, their consulting fee of $12,775 would be due at the end of the introduction period, as well as a $20,000 deposit into a reimbursement account.

Our case specialist offered some dos and don'ts for the dating period. We should talk about our family, friends and hobbies. We should send photos that give a sense for our life, of our surroundings. We should *not* talk about finances, termination or how busy we are.

We were sent Stacey's full profile, which provided more information about who she was, why she wanted to become a surrogate and what kind of relationship she was interested in having. She wrote that she would love to get together once or twice a year but at the very least would love updates and photos a couple times a year. She said she had started talking with her two boys about potentially carrying another baby. Her youngest, she wrote, didn't understand the idea, while her older son was "excited for me to get pregnant and okay with me then giving the baby to another family but would like to see the baby and play with him/her."

Stacey, who works for the provincial government, explained that she had met a surrogate while she was in college and was intrigued at the idea. At the time, she was single and wasn't sure if she could have kids herself. She later experienced a miscarriage before having two sons with her husband, Doug. "They are adorable, smart and hilarious," her profile said, "and I want to give that joy to a couple who can't on their own for one reason or another." She had also loved being pregnant. She liked the attachment she felt, the knowledge that her body was doing this miraculous thing.

She and Doug would lie in bed after their kids went to sleep in the evenings and look through the profiles the agency had sent along. It reminded them of online dating, which is how they met, except now they were looking for a match together. It was more about a feeling they got than about any particular parameter. Knowing that the journey was mostly hers, Stacey wanted Doug to take the lead on choosing the intended parents so he would feel more connected to the process. They initially thought it would be rewarding for Stacey to carry for someone who had experienced miscarriage, as they had themselves. They also thought they would want to help someone who was trying to have their first child.

Our profile and video, though, grabbed them. They were captivated by Sid on the stoop, singing "Mr. Golden Sun." They wanted her to have what their sons had: sibling love.

Dan and I crawled into bed and put the call on speakerphone. My heart was racing, my hands sweaty. We were about to have our first conversation with Stacey and her husband, and we wanted it to go well. We spoke for hours, the conversation flowing and easy. I remember getting off the phone and bursting into tears. "What's wrong?" Dan asked, confused. "I'm just so relieved," I responded, feeling the pressure lift off me. I couldn't believe we were in this situation, but I was starting to believe in the process. I could see it. I could picture it. It didn't seem so unlikely or so unnatural anymore.

The question of trust was top of mind for Stacey too. "I was like, 'How do they trust someone to do this?'" she told me years later. "I would be carrying a part of you—a piece of Dan, a piece of you. And you would have no idea what I'd be doing with my life. You'd be trusting that I'd be eating the right things and taking care of myself, especially given all the money you were pouring into it."

We had been clear with Stacey in that initial call that we still wanted to try one or two more transfers. She said she totally understood and supported whatever we decided; they were our embryos, she said, and we needed to feel 100 percent ready to move on to surrogacy. She wasn't in a rush, she liked us, she was willing to wait. It was a match.

I hadn't been wrong for not trusting my body. Even after another surgery, this time with a gynecological surgeon in the Boston area, my lining remained stubborn and unwilling. On our next transfer cycle, my lining only reached five millimetres but it had a triple-line pattern, so we went ahead with a transfer. It didn't take. We tried a different protocol on the following cycle, but my lining only reached four millimetres and wasn't triple lined, so we cancelled it.

I was comfortable that we had done our best to try to get me viably pregnant. I was comfortable closing this chapter. I was done being the reason we didn't have a baby yet. I was done playing the lead in the sad story of our fertility journey. I was ready for someone fresh and healthy and optimistic to change the narrative. I was ready to move to the periphery and become a supporting member of the cast. I knew it was the right time to make this decision because I felt more relief than anxiety, though the financial stress of moving to surrogacy added a new layer. One woman I spoke with said she could relate to my emotional reaction to moving on to surrogacy after years of treatment. "I remember talking to my therapist, and I was like, 'I'm not sad. I'm done. And I'm going to live my fucking life,'" she said.

Stacey lives in a small town about 150 kilometres northeast of Toronto, so coming to the clinic for screening meant waking up early, arranging for her two kids to get off to daycare or school without her, taking a full day off work and spending several hours in the car. It was the spring of 2021, so the pandemic protocols were still in place; we weren't allowed to accompany her for the initial appointment. The clinic was running late, so she spent the better part of two hours intermittently waiting and getting tests done and waiting some more. We felt terrible about the delays.

That feeling of guilt, of wanting to make things good and okay and easy for her, was immediate and deeply felt. It became clear to me then that there were now three people on this team—four in fact, including her husband. There were other people's emotions, schedules and needs at play. It wasn't just about Dan and me, what we thought and felt, anymore. It was hard to know how to act and be. We had never been intended parents before. Stacey had never been a surrogate before. Maybe that was the beauty of it. We were strangers stumbling through it together.

When Stacey emerged from the clinic, Dan and I were waiting for her on a park bench nearby with some lunch. We didn't hug at first and sat a few metres apart, respecting the public-health restrictions in place. We talked about the testing she'd had done and when we could expect the results. We talked about what our kids had been up to over the previous weekend. We talked about the wraps we were eating. We talked about how work was going and what she had missed to be at the clinic for us that day. When it was time to part ways, I couldn't help but ask if it was okay for me to give her a hug. I felt a compulsion to wrap my arms around her. I cried into her shoulder. I couldn't believe she was real.

"Thank you, thank you, thank you," I whispered.

We didn't know yet if she had passed the medical screening. We still had to sort out legals and pass the mental-health evaluation. But none of that mattered. Whether or not she became our surrogate was immaterial to the mark she had already left on us and our faith in the journey.

Stacey wanted to give us the gift of a child, but she had already given us the gift of hope.

We didn't know much about the surrogacy industry when we began our journey. And it's probably for the best. What I have since come to realize, through our own experience and in my reporting, is enough to give me pause. Because while the surrogacy world is life-giving and features good-hearted, altruistic actors helping to make people's dreams come true, it can also be fraught. There are stories of questionable practices, including the falsification of receipts, the misleading of intended parents about the availability of a prospective surrogate and the luring of surrogates to join an agency with the promise of a free iPad. I've been told that surrogates are sometimes coached by their agencies to squeeze as much as they can from intended parents, including by expensing pricey fitness items they can later resell—a treadmill, for example. I didn't realize until I was doing research into the industry that there are some people in this space who can't stand each other, who won't work with one another.

When Dan and I entered the surrogacy world and chose our agency, CFC, we had felt as though our eyes were open. We were aware that Leia Swanberg had been the first—and, as of this writing, the only—person to be charged and convicted under the federal Assisted Human Reproduction Act. In researching agencies back in 2020, I had come across a 2016 article that ran in *The Globe and Mail*, written by a freelance journalist named Alison Motluk. She has been writing about assisted reproduction for two decades, producing investigative features that have shined a light on the industry's dark corners. Her 2016 *Globe* article described the 2012 police raid of CFC's offices and the subsequent charges that were laid, culminating in Ms. Swanberg and the company paying $60,000 in fines. The story begins like so:

"Her offences," Motluk wrote, "boiled down to paying money to egg donors for their eggs, paying money to surrogates for contract pregnancies and taking finder's fees from an American lawyer who, unbeknownst to Swanberg, was running an elaborate baby-selling ring."

The article went on to say that, according to Swanberg, her business had quadrupled in the years since she was charged. Indeed, we weren't the only ones who were drawn to CFC. After all, it had quoted us the shortest time to a match. For us, and for many others, that simple fact trumped everything. Two fertility lawyers quoted in the *Globe* piece described Swanberg as a champion of surrogates who helps create effective lines of communication between surrogates and intended parents. But Motluk wrote that there were also those who had less flattering things to say, describing Swanberg as "abrasive" and "cruel." "I'm a work-in-progress on that," Swanberg told Motluk at the time. "I definitely lose my shit."

In doing research for this book, I went through the agreed statement of facts in the case against CFC and Swanberg. The case culminated in a plea deal involving three counts: purchasing eggs from donors, paying consideration to surrogates and accepting consideration for arranging the services of a surrogate. It detailed evidence obtained through search warrants and production orders, including financial records, emails and statements gathered from egg donors, surrogates, intended parents, current and former agency staff and Hilary Neiman, a U.S. lawyer convicted in the United States of mail fraud by circumventing adoption laws. (Swanberg told me she accepted a plea deal because she ran out of money to fight the case.)

On count one, the document said that "former and current CFC employees told the RCMP that CFC paid egg donors a flat fee of $5,000 and did not request expense receipts for these payments." It also said that some employees asserted that Swanberg directed them to create "fictitious" or "'estimated' expense spreadsheets." On count two, CFC employees told investigators that the agency paid surrogates the maximum contracted amount for expenses, whether or not the surrogate provided receipts and regardless of what they actually spent.

When it came to count three, the statement of facts referred to the case against Neiman, who, together with two co-accused in the United States, sent surrogates from the United States and Canada to other countries for IVF procedures. "Once pregnancy was confirmed, they sought out intended parents and told them the previous intended parents had backed out of the arrangement," the document said. "In most cases, there were no previous intended parents." The co-accused falsified documents in order to circumvent the adoption process and register the intended parents as legal parents. The statement of facts pointed to three cases in which intended parents were each charged somewhere between $120,000 and $149,000 U.S. for the babies.

In 2011, the statement said, the FBI told the RCMP that Neiman had made payments to Swanberg. The RCMP investigated three occasions on which such payments were paid, totalling $31,000. Neiman told the RCMP these were fees paid in exchange for referrals of intended parents. The statement said, "No record of the U.S. surrogacy agreements were found in CFC files or on its computers, nor were CFC employees aware of these agreements."

The statement of facts also said "the charge against [Swanberg] does not involve any allegation that [Swanberg] defrauded the U.S. government or knowingly or otherwise participated in any such fraud committed by Neiman, but rather that she violated the Canadian regulatory scheme that makes it an offence to accept payment for arranging the services of a surrogate."

Swanberg maintains she didn't know about Neiman's baby-selling scheme, telling me it had been conceivable to her at the time that multiple intended parents could have walked away from their surrogates. Upon reflection, she said she would have asked more questions. "Now I may be more discerning and say 'Prove it,'" she said. "At the time, I saw a solution for clients and offered it to them." As for the illegitimate receipts and expenses, Swanberg said the agency hadn't done enough diligence to ensure surrogates were submitting proper expenses. "We had lots of envelopes with lots of receipts and poor bookkeeping processes," she said. "It wasn't okay to do . . . We took the surrogates at their word and gave them their money."

Dan and I experienced Swanberg's volatility first-hand, her raging phone calls in particular. Years later, I asked her about it. She explained that she had gone through what she described as a mental-health crisis. "I became shitty at work, shitty to people in my life," she said. "My behaviour caused impact for you, and I apologize for that." Swanberg said her actions were always out of a perceived need to protect the surrogates who had signed up to her agency. "I had been so focused—hyper-focused—on the care of the surrogate and the feelings of a surrogate that I have been hard as hell on intended parents," she said. "My intention has always been 'I will get you a kid in a year, if you just do the right things.' Now I realize it's not a race. It's about getting you there gently."

Swanberg told me she has felt demonized and singled out in the media—the easy target of bad press, especially in the wake of the criminal case. She's proud of the work she has done over the years to help people, including Dan and me, find their way to their babies. She was the one, for example, who suggested we reach out to Dr. Daneshmand, the San Diego doctor who consulted on our case. Indeed, there were many conversations where she and the agency supported us. "I can feel really good about that," she said.

It wasn't until after our fertility journey that I fully understood that surrogacy agencies aren't licensed by any level of government. This vacuum, critics say, creates a Wild West in surrogacy, where the stakes are high and the money is flowing. There's a lack of enforcement and accountability. As Motluk wrote in an investigative piece called "Waiting Room," published in literary magazine *Hazlitt* in August 2023, "there are no standards, no requirements, no certifications, no surrogacy-specific licences, and while Health Canada is meant to have the power to audit these organizations, experts say it's not clear that these inspections are actually happening. A surrogacy agency can be anything, and be operated by anyone at all who decides to set one up."

I asked the government about the legal status of surrogacy agencies, which may offer other services but at their core connect surrogates with intended parents. How is what they're doing not considered in breach of the prohibition on arranging the services of a surrogate? Health Canada told me that whether the actions of an agency contravene the act would depend on the specific facts. Only a court, the department said, could make that decision.

"We know that it's illegal to make payment to arrange the services of a surrogate, but we don't know what's considered 'arranging the services,'" Toronto-based fertility lawyer Sara Cohen told me. "If you're going to put people in jail, under criminal law, you better be very clear. And it's not clear." Cohen said it's hard to advise an intended parent to pursue litigation against an agency if they felt they were wronged in some way because of the grey area the agencies operate in. If the intended parent paid the agency and matched with a surrogate, then they could be exposing themselves to legal risk. "Why would you go to sue someone when you could have legal liability?" she said.

Aware of the prohibition on arranging surrogacy services, agencies bill themselves as "consultants" that introduce intended parents to surrogates, who then choose with whom they want to work. They don't *match* people, because they don't make the decision of who gets paired up. CFC, for example, says on its website that its role is to "introduce surrogates to couples or individuals who need help fulfilling their dreams of parenthood" and to "provide guidance and support throughout the rest of the process." There's no mention of arranging for the service of the surrogate. Swanberg said roughly 10 percent of intended parents who connect with a surrogate through the agency end up taking that relationship and leaving without paying the considerable "consulting fee," which is collected after the parties agree to match.

Another agency, Surrogacy in Canada Online, flags on its site that it's illegal to pay an individual to arrange the services of a surrogate. "We cannot guarantee or 'match' you with a surrogate," the site says. "Surrogates choose which intended parents they wish to match with." Surrogacy in Canada Online has been around a long time—since 2001, a few years before the federal act came into play. Founder Sally Rhoads-Heinrich said to ensure her agency wasn't breaking the law as it relates to accepting payment for arranging the services of a surrogate, she created a membership model with an online portal for surrogates and intended parents to connect themselves. Intended parents pay $8,500 to join (as of early 2025), without any guarantee of a match. The ratios are always changing, Rhoads-Heinrich said. There are typically somewhere between one and ten surrogates available and somewhere in the order of sixty intended parents. Unlike CFC, Surrogacy in Canada Online doesn't manage the payment of expenses.

"It's frustrating that hairdressers and taxi drivers have to have a licence but surrogacy consultants don't," said Rhoads-Heinrich, who has herself been a surrogate. "That's why I don't manage the money . . . We're not banks. I don't want to touch it."

This hands-off approach to managing expenses might bring comfort to intended parents who are worried about transferring large sums of money to an agency for disbursement to surrogates. Reimbursement funds in Canada, after all, aren't required to be held in trust. If the agency goes under, the money is gone. And technically, there's nothing stopping an agency from using the money to make payroll and then praying it has enough funds to reimburse its surrogates when the time comes. There have been some alarming cases of companies in the United States making off with their clients' money. A 2024 lawsuit, for example, accuses the owner of a Houston escrow company, which was supposed to be holding money in trust, of stealing millions of dollars from intended parents to fund her music career and take lavish trips.

I spoke with someone in Canada who didn't go the agency route to find a surrogate because, as a lawyer herself, she was concerned about the legal ambiguity. If she and her husband, also a lawyer, paid an agency to help them find a surrogate, could they potentially be found guilty of breaking the law? They were worried about losing their licences to practise law and in turn their livelihoods. "We read the Assisted Human Reproduction Act," she said, "and we were both like, 'Hmmm.'"

The ban on commercial surrogacy in Canada is rooted in the idea that the government should prohibit the commodification of the female body. It's also meant to discourage a woman from becoming a surrogate for financial reasons. In this line of thinking, women—particularly those who are vulnerable for financial or mental-health reasons—need to be protected against exploitation, including by coercive third parties.

Dara Roth Edney, a social worker who founded her Informed Fertility counselling practice in 2007, had two daughters through surrogacy. One was born before the 2004 act outlawing compensation, and the other was born after. Roth Edney said she and her husband insisted on paying their first surrogate, as was allowed at the time. Although it was a deeply personal relationship, Roth Edney said it was important to her that the surrogate be recognized for her hard work and literal labour. As for her second surrogate, after the new rules came in, Roth Edney and her husband sent her flowers on her birthday, purchased small gifts for her children and gave her a necklace with their daughter's birthstone after the delivery.

I asked her why she felt comfortable sharing this with me, given the law. "Maybe I'm wrong and I'm going to the big house, but I cannot fathom a scenario in which a Crown attorney could convince a court that my surrogate was a vulnerable woman who never would have done this save for the compensation—when the compensation was flowers on her birthday and stuffed animals for her children on Christmas," she said. "Nobody is putting their bodies through this because you bought them flowers or a pretty necklace."

Even when intended parents are doing their absolute best to remain within the letter of the law, the rules on reimbursement were for years vague. There has long been confusion about what constitutes a legitimate expense. What about a surrogate's monthly phone bill? After all, she needs to regularly communicate with the intended parents. What about a surrogate's mortgage payment? It's important that the surrogate have a reliable place to live. What about a spa treatment? It's important the surrogate isn't overly stressed. A gym membership? Staying active can contribute to the health of the surrogate and the baby.

In 2020, sixteen years after commercial surrogacy was criminalized under the Assisted Human Reproduction Act, the federal government released regulations outlining what expenses are allowed under the law. The list includes, but isn't limited to, expenditures for transportation, the care of dependants or pets, counselling, maternity clothes, telecommunications, groceries and prenatal exercise classes. The regulations don't provide a minimum or maximum amount for each category. For example, when it comes to groceries, the idea is that pregnant people generally eat more than they consumed when not pregnant. Practically speaking, though, how much more is the "right" amount of more? Unclear. One lawyer put it to me this way: If an intended parent is confused about whether a surrogate's expense is legally reimbursable, they can apply the *but for* test. *But for her being pregnant, would she incur this expense?* If the answer is no, the expense is likely legitimate. The idea is that a surrogate shouldn't be out of pocket for expenses associated with helping someone have a baby.

Swanberg said she sees nothing wrong with explaining to surrogates how they can maximize what they get reimbursed for. She used the example of a litter box. For medical reasons, a pregnant woman shouldn't handle cat litter, so if the surrogate has to pay someone to come to their home and do that chore for them, she should have every right to do so and to expense that cost.

The ban on paying for surrogacy in Canada is also controversial because everyone is getting paid except the surrogates—the fertility doctors, the pharmaceutical companies, the lawyers, social workers, agencies et cetera. "Oftentimes, the [surrogate's] husband or the partner doesn't want the surrogate to go through with a journey if they're not going to get paid for it," Rhoads-Heinrich said. She went on to explain that surrogates aren't out for huge salaries but are oftentimes looking for a way to stay home with their own children. "The number one surrogate candidate is a woman coming off a one-year maternity leave; they're not ready to send their kid to daycare," she said. "But many withdraw from the application process once they find out it's not paid."

It can be particularly hard, she explained, for domestic intended parents to compete with international intended parents, who in some cases are courting Canadian surrogates with financial compensation. Seeing themselves at a significant disadvantage, some intended parents in Canada have expanded their search to countries such as the United States and Mexico. One intended parent in Canada wrote on a surrogacy Facebook page that she was three years into a search for a surrogate—with no luck, she said, because of what she described as competition from high-paying international intended parents. She said the landscape in Canada had become hopeless.

The Canadian Fertility and Andrology Society has for years said the criminalization of commercial surrogacy and gamete donation severely limits the number of surrogates and donors in Canada. Those in need, the society has pointed out, includes not just infertile people but also cancer patients, same-sex couples and single would-be parents. The society proposed that the federal government amend the act to allow for what it describes as "reasonable compensation" of donors and surrogates.

One fertility lawyer I spoke with said the prohibition on paying surrogates and the legal penalties for contravening the law is paternalistic and misdirected. "We're hard-wired as a species to reproduce, on top of all the societal norms and expectations," the lawyer said. "It's Darwinian. To not be able to accomplish that, there's desperation, anxiety, suicidal ideation, relationship breakdowns. And then to turn these people into criminals because there isn't a friend or relative to help them, it's preposterous. Further, it creates a vulnerable population ripe for exploiting."

Cindy Wasser, the founder and principal lawyer of Hope Springs Fertility Law who acted on behalf of Dan and me, said she interprets the law such that there is nothing explicitly barring intended parents from paying their surrogate *after* she has delivered and parentage has been established. "The handing over of custody brings her back to being a woman, not a surrogate, and there's nothing preventing you from giving a woman anything you want," she said.

Health Canada didn't respond directly to my question about Ms. Wasser's interpretation of the law. The department said determining whether paying a surrogate contravenes prohibitions set out in the act depends on the specific facts of the situation. Again, Health Canada said only a court can ultimately decide whether the law has been broken.

From a pure economics perspective, the bottom line is that people are willing to do the work and people are willing to pay. Proponents of a compensation model argue that regulations could be introduced to establish rates and an upper cap. Proponents of maintaining the altruistic model say they understand that compensation is a way of demonstrating gratitude, but they worry it could open a can of worms. Should surrogates get danger pay for carrying twins, for example? The decriminalization of paying surrogates, Cattapan said, might create a situation that's "a little too *Handmaid's Tale* for everybody"—a reference to the Margaret Atwood novel in which women are forced to produce children for the ruling class. Compared to other jurisdictions, she said, Canada's system is "working pretty well." The country, she said, is seen as an ethical destination for surrogacy.

University of Ottawa professor Vanessa Gruben, the principal investigator on the Surrogates' Voices project, said surrogates had mixed views on the prohibition on compensation but overall didn't support the idea of a free market for surrogacy. "There was a strong consensus that Canada should not move to an unregulated paid system," she said. I asked Stacey what she thought about the ban on paying surrogates. She said she supported the law. "I didn't want to feel like I was selling my body," she said. "I wanted to give the gift of a first child or a sibling."

As for intended parents, I spoke with one woman who told me she would have preferred to have agreed with her surrogate on a lump sum payment at the outset. Instead, the surrogate who carried her first child "maxed out her expenses every month and charged for crazy things," including a laptop, an unfathomable amount of chocolate, groceries and takeout every day for her entire family and hundreds of dollars of maternity clothes each and every month. It was unpredictable and grating. "By this point, she was growing my baby and I had no power," the woman said. She was desperate. "I thought, 'She's got your baby. Just shut up and pay it.'"

And while there are stories about surrogates pushing the limits of what should be expensed, there are also stories of intended parents pushing back too far. The classic example I have heard is an intended parent questioning their surrogate over an appointment-related parking fee: *Couldn't you have parked further from the clinic and gotten a cheaper spot?*

The Canadian approach to surrogacy lies in contrast with the landscape south of the border, where surrogates in many states are paid a salary, usually somewhere in the order of $60,000 to $100,000 U.S., depending on a number of factors, including where they live and whether they're a first-time surrogate or have experience. One could argue that surrogates in these cases are less likely to be or feel exploited. To guard against the coercion of surrogates, agencies in the United States disqualify a potential gestational carrier if the person receives any form of government assistance. There are also boutique surrogacy agencies in the United States that offer tiered packages with express options that expedite the time to a match, at a cost upward of half a million dollars.

Oftentimes, those who own or work at surrogacy agencies were surrogates themselves. Take, for example, Alexandra Ryan, who carried for celebrity couple Chrissy Teigen and John Legend and who now works for a U.S. agency as an intake coordinator. In 2020, Teigen suffered a public late-term loss of a baby who would have been her third child. The couple decided to look for a surrogate to potentially carry their future child and, with the help of an agency, found Ryan. They immediately clicked over video call, Ryan told me. When it came time to meet in person at the couple's home, though, she was self-conscious. "I didn't even want to sit on their furniture," she said. "I was like, 'I'm too poor to sit on this.' And Chrissy was like, 'Please, just sit down.'"

Teigen ended up undergoing an embryo transfer and getting pregnant before Ryan did an embryo transfer herself. That transfer stuck, too, so the women were pregnant together and gave birth about five months apart. They went to OB appointments together, they craved Jack in the Box tacos together and their families spent time together. "Chrissy was very 'Eat what you want, give in to your cravings, because I'm doing the same,'" she said. "My daughter thought their house was basically Disneyland—the toys, the big backyard. I remember losing track of her for a few minutes and then found her playing on the piano. I was like, 'Not my daughter going for John Legend's piano.' I almost had a heart attack."

Ryan gave birth to Teigen and Legend's fourth child in June 2023. The couple named the baby boy Wren Alexander, after Alexandra.

Our own journey, thankfully, was moving along. Stacey was medically cleared by Hannam, her lining having achieved a fluffy nine millimetres with a clear triple-line pattern. She and her husband also had a psychological screening session with a counsellor who specializes in fertility. Unsurprisingly to us, Stacey and Doug—both hard-working, responsible, kind and reliable people—were cleared to move forward. We deposited the first $20,000 installment into our reimbursement account and signed our clinic's consent form regarding the use of a gestational carrier.

The twenty-three-page document, which Stacey also signed, outlined the surrogacy process and the risks that treatment could pose. In reading through the risks of pregnancy for the gestational carrier, I was amazed that women sign up for this: miscarriage, ectopic pregnancy, hypertension/pre-eclampsia, gestational diabetes, infection, premature labour, C-section, postpartum depression and anxiety, and death. The overall mortality rate associated with pregnancy, the consent form stated, is 0.01 percent, or one in ten thousand. Of course, one in ten thousand is extremely rare, but still, Stacey was enlisting for something riskier than not signing up for it. And she was incurring these risks for *us*.

We also moved forward with drafting a legal agreement, at a cost of roughly $7,000 in lawyers' fees. The thirty-eight-page agreement stated that Dan and I would be the legal, custodial and social parents of the child and that Stacey and her husband waived any and all rights to the child. It also laid out the circumstances under which either party could terminate the agreement.

There were the obvious stipulations. Among them: If the pregnancy is deemed to pose a "serious risk" to the surrogate's health or life, the surrogate can choose to terminate; immediately upon birth, Stacey would give over the child to us as the custodians; we would only transfer one embryo at a time; the surrogate would follow the treating physician's medical instructions; if a pregnancy didn't result within three transfers, either party could terminate the agreement; we would keep each other reasonably informed of our whereabouts throughout treatment and any ensuing pregnancy; Stacey won't smoke or drink during pregnancy.

And the less obvious ones: During pregnancy, Stacey "shall not knowingly ingest any food or beverage which contains aspartame or any other sugar substitute"; she will not "knowingly ingest foods, beverages or medications which contain caffeine in excess of 300 milligrams per day in the aggregate"; she will not have any part of her body pierced or tattooed; "upon 48-hours' notice, the surrogate and the spouse will make their home available to a representative of Canadian Fertility Consulting for visits prior to the transfer and during the pregnancy"; the surrogate will not travel outside Canada after twenty-four weeks gestation and will not travel more than a sixty-minute drive from a hospital after the end of the thirty-fourth week of pregnancy.

The parts of the agreement dealing with termination were enough to cause even the chillest intended parent some anxiety. In Canada, a person has full and total control over their body. What that means in the context of surrogacy is that if, for example, the intended parents want to terminate a pregnancy because in-utero tests detected genetic or congenital abnormalities or defects, the surrogate does not, under the law, need to have an abortion. If the surrogate continues with the pregnancy and a child is born with the defect, the intended parents can abandon the baby to the child-welfare system. If the child is born without the defect, the surrogate must agree to turn the baby over to the intended parents.

The opposite is also true. If the surrogate wants to abort the pregnancy at any time for any reason, she has the right to do so. "The parties acknowledge that the surrogate has the right in her sole discretion, to have the pregnancy terminated at any time she determines the pregnancy should be terminated," our agreement said. "However, the surrogate has assured the genetic parents that it is not her intention to exercise her right to terminate the pregnancy except in the circumstances described in [sections of the agreement dealing with the health and well-being of the unborn child or the surrogate]."

Wasser, the fertility lawyer, told me about a file she had just worked on involving a surrogate who got pregnant for a married couple abroad. When the surrogate was seven weeks, the intended parents asked her to have an abortion because they were having marital problems, in large part due to the husband's mental health, and were planning to split up. At this stage of gestation, the surrogate likely could have taken the abortion pill. The surrogacy agreement had stipulated that the surrogate would terminate the pregnancy for medical reasons, but there was no such medical reason in this case. Understandably, the surrogate was very upset and sought guidance from her surrogacy agency, which, Wasser said, encouraged the surrogate to resist having an abortion. The surrogate carried the pregnancy to term and the intended parents, who were "semi-together" and had sought counselling, took custody of the baby.

Wasser had a nightmarish surrogacy journey of her own in 2008 in the lead-up to the birth of her first child. She told me about the challenges she faced, namely communication that became so sporadic that she and her husband hired a private investigator to track down the surrogate, whom they had met on Craigslist. Wasser believes the psychological assessments that surrogates undergo ahead of a journey fail to adequately screen for red flags because they don't dive deep enough. She hasn't seen or spoken to the surrogate since the day she signed the parentage documents. When it came time to give her daughter a sibling, Wasser turned to CFC for help.

Entering into a surrogacy agreement also requires that all parties have an up-to-date will in place, including provisions around a testamentary guardian for the unborn child in the event of the death of the intended parents during the pregnancy. And what if, God forbid, the surrogate is rendered incapacitated or requires life support? Whomever is listed in her will as her agent or decision-maker would have power over her medical care. "However, it is the express wish of the surrogate that if she is pregnant with the child at the time of such an incident, and the attending physician deems that the child would benefit from prolonging the life of the surrogate by artificial means until it is deemed safe to deliver the child, the agent or decision maker will prolong the life of the surrogate by artificial means until after the birth of the child," the contract said.

I remember sitting on our bedroom floor at the cottage, going over the agreement on Dan's computer while Sid played outside with her cousins. We could hear her laughing through the cracked-open window. We felt so far from hearing the giggle of our second child. I had to almost disassociate from the legalese in the agreement, else it all felt too scary, too overwhelming. I closed my eyes and hung onto the sound of Sid's laughter. It was innocent and unencumbered. It reminded me to let go.

Either Way

WHEN IT CAME time for Stacey to attempt her first transfer in the spring of 2021, we were all feeling the hope and anticipation. We had several genetically balanced embryos. We had a healthy uterus.

The three of us had lunch at a park together after the transfer, chatting about anything other than the potential pregnancy but thinking only of it. When it was time to part ways, we hugged goodbye. It hit me then that our child might actually grow outside my body. It would hear Stacey's voice, feel her heartbeat, move through *her* life, *her* world. It would move *through* her, *in* her. I wasn't sad, but I wasn't not sad. I was . . . discombobulated. I, of course, knew the plan was to have Stacey grow our baby, but now the seed was actually trying to take root. I kept my feet planted firmly in the mantra my friend had imparted: The goal is baby in arms.

We kept in close touch with Stacey over the next few days, checking in on how she was feeling. The nine-day wait was easier for me than it was in transfers prior; I wasn't reading into every sensation within my body, hoping it was a sign of life. It was also harder in a different way. We had all agreed Stacey would not take any pregnancy tests before the ninth day, because it can provide a false negative. Still, Dan and I read into every text she sent. If we didn't hear from her for a few hours, we would spiral, assume the worst—she had peed on a stick and was processing the bad news, mustering the strength to tell us. In reality, she was playing with her boys or making dinner or not attached to her phone the way Dan and I were.

We woke up on the ninth day post-transfer, knowing Stacey would pee on a stick that morning and we would have our answer. I opened my eyes at an ungodly hour and couldn't fall back to sleep. Hours later, I got a text from Stacey. "Unfortunately, I have some disappointing news this morning," she wrote. "Test read not pregnant. I'm sorry guys. I've been thinking of how to tell you for the last hour and a half, but there is no way to make this less painful to hear."

My heart sank and rose into my throat the way it always did when we got bad fertility news. My eyes welled with tears the way they always did. I told Dan. He probably said something like "fuck" or "what the fuck." We hugged the way we always did when we got information like this. We kissed the way we always did. We had too much experience with bad news to be shocked by it anymore.

"It's okay, Stacey!" I responded. "We know how these things work. And it's really just a matter of luck, at the end of the day . . . We really don't want you to feel badly. We're a team, and we lost the first game. That's all."

"I know we all knew it was a possibility, but it's just really disappointing," she wrote back.

"Of course it's disappointing, but we're gonna keep our chins up," I replied. "Love you."

"Love you, too," she wrote.

Bloodwork confirmed the transfer didn't work. And the hits kept coming. By hits, I mean life. Regular shmegular life. One of Stacey's sons gave her a hard time that night going to bed, testing her patience. Sid got carsick on the way back into the city and puked everywhere.

We pulled over so we could strip her down and clean up. Sid, barefoot and naked with vomit in her hair, picked flowers on the side of the highway. All we could do was laugh.

It had been a year and a half since we had started IVF, and more than two years since our first miscarriage trying to make our second child. By this time, my sister had had her second baby. She called us a few hours after delivering. They hadn't known the sex. It turned out to be a baby girl, the daughter of her dreams, a sister to her son. I remember Dan and I taking the video call and congratulating her and then taking turns crying in the bathroom while the other finished sitting with Sid for her dinner. Most of my closest friends had already had their second babies. Even the friend who was about to start IVF after a near-fatal ectopic pregnancy had just days before given birth to a baby she managed to conceive naturally. We were happy for them and also jealous.

Stacey was ready to try again as soon as possible, so when she started her period, she called in her day one for her next transfer, resumed the estrogen patches, drove into Toronto for a lining check, got the green light to start progesterone and was given a transfer date. Stacey came into the city on transfer day with her husband and two sons. We had made plans to have lunch afterward in our backyard, the seven of us, and get to know each other better, introduce the kids. It was a hot summer day, so Dan set up the sprinkler and some water toys in the back. Sid, at this point three and a half years old, greeted their family with a smile, having no idea who they were or why they were at our house. We told her they were our friends over for a lunch date and playtime. Our reason for being coy with her was about protecting her heart, and ours.

Sid had been starting to notice the world around her more and more—the bigger, louder, busier families, the babies, the siblings holding hands on their way to school. She would sporadically ask why she wasn't a big sister, like this person or that person. We would tell her that families come in all different sizes, that not everyone has a brother or sister. There were times she would come up to me, lift my shirt and ask if there was a baby in my tummy. On one such occasion, I was in the middle of a miscarriage. A pad soaking up blood in my underwear, I got down on my knees, looked into her blue eyes and said, "No, sweetheart." And then, like so many women in the midst of a loss, I went to the kitchen and made dinner.

I had become hypersensitive to the idea that she was conscious of not having a sibling. Everything she said or did became coded. I could see reminders everywhere. I would go to the dentist and the medical form would ask if I was pregnant or breastfeeding. I would fill out an online registration form for a program for Sid and a drop-down menu would give the option to enroll siblings at the same time. I would see the storage bins of all the clothes and shoes and toys and gear she had grown out of, wondering if we would ever get to use them again. They were piling up, towering over us, taunting us. I would see the maternity jeans folded in my closet.

Every now and then, Sid would pull out a faded and flimsy Berenstain Bears book from her bookshelf, and I would feel my chest tighten.

Brother Bear. Sister Bear. Baby Bear.

Brother. Sister. Baby.

So fearful of highlighting the thing she was missing out on as a Baum kid, I found myself renaming the characters: Older Bear, Younger Bear and Youngest Bear. I was terrified of stirring something in her. I don't know why I didn't hide those books. I should have. I should have done a better job protecting my heart in these small ways, because the small things add up, chip away at your resilience. They feel big and they make you tired.

I'm sure a lot of it was in my head, but at the time it felt entirely real and entirely soul-crushing. I felt like we were depriving her of something meaningful. I had to remind myself that we were all healthy, that her needs were provided for, that life was good. *Life is good* became one of my key mantras, alongside *Calm is my superpower.* I wanted to achieve equanimity, move through life unmoved. Not numb, but not rattled.

And so I watched Sid giggle with Stacey's sons as they stuck out their tongues to lap up the water shooting from our sprinkler that summer day after the transfer. I took deep breaths. I smiled. I quieted the voice in my head that worried it was too hot outside for the embryo to properly implant. I let thoughts pass by like clouds floating across the sky.

The next week managed to move along. I wouldn't say it flew by, because time never does in the post-transfer nine-day waiting window, but it wasn't as paralyzing as it had been in transfers past. Stacey, for her part, was struggling to stay present. "Feeling really anxious today," she wrote me. "Halfway through this waiting period and just really want this one to take."

A couple of days before the scheduled bloodwork to determine whether the transfer worked, I received a text from Stacey.

"I feel absolutely horrible, don't know why it doesn't want to stick. They say everything looks good and I have no problem with natural conception, but the transfers are not going as I hoped and I'm doing everything that I've always done when we were trying to get pregnant or were pregnant. Very frustrating for me as I feel like I want this as much as you guys do, if that is even possible. I'm sooo sorry."

This was something Stacey had wanted to do for someone for over a decade, and now it was taking over her life just as it had ours.

I couldn't help but think we were robbing her of her dream to carry someone else's baby. She shouldn't have picked us.

Because Dan and I were both working from home at this point, bad news travelled fast. It was dinnertime when the text came in. We were in the kitchen, feeding Sid her meal and preparing our own. "It's Stacey," I said. I shook my head. "Bad news," I said, matter of fact. I handed him my phone and took over sitting with Sid. He read the message and let out a long exhale. He does this thing whenever his frustration mounts to a point that's hard to contain, where he punches his right fist into the open palm of his left hand and lets out a primal grunt. He did that. We wrapped our arms around each other as Sid continued to eat her dinner, careful not to crumble in front of her.

Unsurprisingly, Thursday's bloodwork came back negative. No one knew why. Not our doctor. Not our nurse. Not anyone else we consulted. We'll never know why those two transfers didn't take. One thing was for damn sure: We had struggled with recurrent miscarriage, and now we were grappling with repeated implantation failure.

"Since IVF started almost fifty years ago, we've come so far with what we can do—genetic screening, medications et cetera," said Dr. Sierra, the reproductive endocrinologist in Toronto. "But the black box . . . is what happens with implantation. Implantation is this amazing symphony that allows an embryo to attach. There's so much we don't know, including when it comes to recurrent implantation failure. We generate beautiful embryos in the lab and then time and time again they don't take."

The bottom line is that if you can afford to persist, financially and emotionally, you could well end up with a baby. As Dr. Sierra put it, "Keep going. Take care of yourselves. Keep going."

With a master's in psychology, Dr. Sierra has a broad view of the patient experience. Her thesis was on the internal locus of control, and it's proved a helpful lens in relating to people going through recurrent loss or recurrent implantation failure. "There's a theory that when you can internalize control and be in charge of your environment, it's a psychologically happier place to be," she said. "It's difficult to thrive when you're not the master of your domain. When you're at the fertility clinic, control is out the window. It's a hard place to be. I'm struck by how strong people are, every single day."

In July 2021, Dr. Hannam suggested that we run a funded retrieval cycle—that we make more embryos, given that we only had one left and given our story thus far. We probably had one or two more transfers with Stacey before one of us said it was time to move on. With more embryos, it would give us the opportunity to select the highest-quality one for our next transfer. Also, if we transferred that last embryo into Stacey and it didn't work, we would be caught flat-footed, with no embryos, on Stacey's following cycle.

We had put our name on Hannam's waitlist for a provincially subsidized cycle when we signed on at the clinic. We'd hoped we wouldn't need to access the funding by the time we became eligible for it. But here we were, knee-deep in IVF fees, with no baby, stressing about the financial implications of surrogacy. "I do think it's time," Dr. Hannam wrote to us. "We have a spot if you feel ready."

I broke down in tears at the idea of giving my body over to IVF again. But I didn't give myself the option of saying no. Forging ahead was still a matter of course. And if I was going to do it, I wanted to get on with it.

As for the next transfer with Stacey, Dr. Hannam agreed with two other doctors we'd consulted, who had said that we should do a different transfer protocol that more closely mimics the body's natural release of hormones. The upside to a modified natural transfer cycle is that it's associated with slightly higher pregnancy rates in patients with normal cycles. The downside is that it requires more monitoring, which means more clinic visits, more commuting into the city, more disruption and unpredictability.

Stacey was gearing up for a transfer, and I was gearing up for a retrieval. Two women, arm in arm, fixated on the goal of a baby. If this next transfer didn't work, there may be a future without Stacey. We had no idea what that would look like.

The lead-up to the retrieval was, yet again, hellish. On a whack of hormones, I grew dozens of eggs—a good problem to have, I knew, but a horrible feeling. My estradiol was through the roof. It had risen so high that Dr. Hannam was concerned enough to call me himself. I was in bed in the middle of the day when he rang to suggest that we trigger a bit earlier than in cycles past and that we forgo the hCG shot altogether. Avoiding hCG would reduce my chances of developing severe OHSS.

My hormones responded to the trigger medication as they should, so we moved ahead with the retrieval. I was put under conscious sedation, Dan provided his sample and Dr. Hannam extracted thirty eggs. I woke up groggy, went home, continued the high salt diet, felt better than I had after previous retrievals. The lab advised us that the retrieval yielded seventeen mature eggs, eleven of which fertilized normally. But as the days passed, only three embryos survived to the biopsy stage and were frozen. In the end, one came back genetically normal.

The results raised the possibility of a fourth retrieval. Doctors generally advise against doing egg retrievals back to back, as your body (chiefly your ovaries) needs time to reset. We had received bad news on so many occasions that we felt vulnerable with only the one embryo slated to be transferred into Stacey in the coming days, plus the single embryo we had just made. It didn't feel like enough.

The transfer into Stacey proceeded as the other two had. The embryo hatched nicely; her lining looked great. The transfer was more likely to work than it was to fail; the law of probabilities told us so. And the stakes felt higher than ever. We were worried it would be our last transfer with Stacey—that if it didn't work, she would be done with us. Her husband had been suffering from severe back pain and had just been diagnosed with an illness that required prolonged treatment. We figured we were a burden they would want to shed.

We asked her not to test until the end of the upcoming weekend, as we had family plans, including my brother's fortieth birthday, and we wanted to enjoy ourselves as best we could. And then Sunday morning came. It was 7:04 a.m. when her text came in.

Words.

Words.

Words.

Negative.

Words.

I sat up in bed and cried into the white duvet cover.

I screamed into my pillow.

I rolled over and buried my face into Dan's chest.

I read the rest of the message through my blurry tears. "I am so frustrated and annoyed," Stacey wrote. "Every time I have to tell you this, it gets harder and harder."

She felt guilty that it wasn't working. What a wild dynamic. I spoke about this with a friend of mine, Tim, who has two children with his husband. He told me about their journey—about how they fertilized half of their donor's eggs with his sperm and the other half with that of his husband. That way, they could both have a shot at biological children. When it came time to decide whose embryo should go first for a transfer into their surrogate, they decided they didn't want to "play God." And so, with the surrogate's consent, they transferred two embryos: one of his and one of his husband's. Both of the embryos stuck. They were having twins. But within a couple of weeks, they lost one of the pregnancies.

"Our surrogate felt horrible," Tim recalled. "I remember sitting in the waiting room afterward, rubbing her back and reassuring her because she felt so bad." It was a case of what's known as vanishing twin syndrome, in which one of the embryos stops developing and is then absorbed by the pregnant woman and the surviving embryo. Ever since he told me about this, I've been thinking about this idea of absorption, about how his surrogate took on his loss. She was changed, at a cellular level.

Stacey told us she was headed to the cottage with her husband to celebrate their anniversary and take some time to themselves, to check out and disconnect. We spoke upon their return, commiserating about the intractability of it all. Stacey said she understood if we wanted to "break up" with her and find another surrogate but also said she was up for doing another transfer if we wanted to try again.

I was entirely daunted at the thought of finding another surrogate. It wasn't just about the search. It was also about forging a relationship again, developing trust. I couldn't imagine trusting someone the way I had grown to trust Stacey. I couldn't imagine starting over again, getting through the awkward phase of committing to something so intensely intimate with someone we didn't know. It felt like a bridge too far, a mountain too steep.

It was at this stage in the process that I began to waver, to feel the lure of surrender. I wasn't saying that I was done, but I was saying that I wasn't all in. I raised the possibility of transferring our last embryo into Stacey. What would be would be. If nothing came of that, we could be done.

It felt like a crazy thing to say out loud, given the time, energy and money we had poured into our quest thus far. But it was also entirely sane. It had by that point been two years since we had started IVF. Sid's fourth birthday was around the corner. When was enough,

enough? Had the time come? I knew something had shifted in me because I no longer felt sad. I felt angry. Not that we weren't pregnant yet. Not that we didn't have a second child. I was pissed off that we weren't letting ourselves live our lives with arms wide open, that we weren't allowing ourselves the luxury of making plans and keeping them, that we weren't giving our daughter the gift of being present and joyful. I was sick of wishing away time when I had no business doing so. I was resenting the journey more than I was committed to seeing it through. I had opened my mind to the possibility—the probability, even—of having one child. For months, I had gone by the mantra *One day, one way.* But I had started to despise those words. My mantra became *It will happen or it won't, and either way we will be happy.* I had to start letting go, even if we kept going. It wasn't necessarily about doing less; it was about letting less of the pain in.

Anything I did from that point forward was exclusively for Dan and Sid; I wasn't doing it for me anymore. I was picturing life with Sid, the three of us. And it felt good. It felt right. It felt full. I let myself feel how I was feeling, without judgment, and I realized that I didn't *need* another baby the way I thought I did. I could be happy with "just one." I *was* happy with one.

Dara Roth Edney, the fertility counsellor, said she has seen this sort of evolution in perspective among her own patients. "Sometimes, people get so worn down by the trauma of the fertility journey that something happens that makes them say, 'Do I even want a baby? Is it worth all of this?'" she said. "At the start, you feel like you'll go to the end of the earth, you'll do whatever you need to do because you have the hope of a baby. Over time, you can't see the baby anymore. All you can see is the trauma. It starts to feel like all you're doing is hurting yourself, to no end. That ambivalence isn't about not wanting a baby anymore. It's that the pain is so huge that a baby doesn't feel possible."

It can be hard for those people, she said, to decide to find their limit. I asked if there's also an element of pride and perfectionism that comes into play. "People are often so used to trying and fighting that they don't know what else to do," she said. "You've invested so much into having a baby—your effort, your money. You've focused on that to the detriment of your work and your relationships. How can you let go without a baby?" It doesn't help, she said, that we live in a world that judges stopping as failure. "There's all the Instagrammers who say 'Never give up,'" she said. "But stopping something that's causing you pain is not giving up."

Dan was in an entirely different headspace than I was. The more obstacles that came our way, the more stubborn and fixated he became, the more he dug in. He assured me that his persistence was motivated by the pure desire for another child, not by some ego-driven mission to "win" the game of fertility. He visibly recoiled when I suggested that we might soon be done with all this, that we might not get what we want because you don't always get what you want in life. We all have a cross to bear. No one has cancer. *Life is good.*

I could see he wasn't ready to call it. After we put Sid to bed one night, we sat down in the family room and had an honest conversation about where we were at and what might come next. It was the first time we conceded that the next steps weren't presumed. "If we're going to try to find another surrogate, you'll need to take the lead," I told him. "I will do another retrieval," I said, as if I was doing him a favour, "but I cannot fathom finding another surrogate. I just don't have it in me, not right now."

Dan took the reins firmly in his own two hands and proceeded to send a flurry of emails. To the doctor in San Diego for another opinion on our file. To a second Canadian surrogacy agency we had signed up with months ago, so we could get a sense for where we were in their queue. To a U.S. surrogacy agency to learn what doing a journey south of the border would look like. To our team at

Hannam to ask if they could look at my lining to be sure it hadn't magically improved. (It hadn't.) To our surrogacy agency to let them know we were looking to start the process of finding another surrogate. CFC told us it would take somewhere in the order of six months to be rematched through traditional means. That was too long. There had to be another way.

Our contact at CFC suggested we try what they called a "rematch hack"—a self-directed, social-media approach that several intended parents in our situation had apparently used with great success. It involved creating a Meta Business page on Facebook that asked for help finding a surrogate and then paying to boost the content, as if it was an ad. That way, it had a better chance of being seen by target audiences, namely females aged twenty-five to thirty-eight living in Canada with certain tagged interests. It felt strange to put ourselves out there in this way. Seeing the photos of Sid's smiling, innocent face on the page felt almost exploitive. We were trying to get people's attention, wanted to pull at their heartstrings. We had to put our pride and discomfort aside.

We heard from women pretty much immediately. One of them told us she had been about to do a transfer for a couple in Italy when COVID hit, derailing the journey. Her messages with Dan sounded promising, but when it came to setting up a time to speak, she was unreliable. One woman sounded great but was unvaccinated against COVID. Another had six cats. I remembered from *Expecting Better* that kitty litter can be a potential source of toxoplasmosis, a type of parasitic infection that can pass across the placenta to the baby, potentially causing serious neurological complications. It's not as if women with cats shouldn't get pregnant, but they do need to be very careful. This wasn't a layer of risk we were willing to assume.

As we messaged with potential surrogates over Facebook, we pretty quickly figured out which questions to ask up front. Some were more personal than others, so there was a cadence to the conversations that built up to the more sensitive queries. Had she been a surrogate before? Had she had at least one live birth? Was she married or in a serious relationship? Did she have a strong support network? Is she on any medications? Is she vaccinated against COVID-19? Does she smoke, drink or do any drugs? Does she get regular periods? It was odd to get so intimate with people so quickly, but it was also par for the course and entirely necessary. There were also some common questions the women asked of us. Did we already have embryos? How long does it usually take from the time we match till the first transfer? What kind of relationship did we foresee during the pregnancy? After the birth?

At the same time as we were pushing forward on the surrogacy front, we were moving ahead with another egg retrieval. I always looked forward to the actual procedure. I so adored that soothing, soaring twilight sedation. I arrived at the clinic over Thanksgiving weekend and was told that a different doctor would be doing the retrieval, which made me uncomfortable, but there was nothing to be done.

The doctor retrieved about half as many eggs as Dr. Hannam had in retrievals past. When I was lucid later that day, I emailed Dr. Hannam with our concerns, apologizing for the intrusion on the long weekend. Apologizing as if I was somehow unreasonable for feeling uneasy that a different doctor had done the procedure, for feeling confused by the disparity in the number of eggs extracted.

I remember Dan crawling into bed beside me that night. I remember him putting his arm around me. I remember dozing back off. I remember, hours later, needing to use the washroom. I remember sitting on the edge of the bed, knowing I shouldn't stand up too fast, knowing I had felt faint from the medications in the days and weeks prior, knowing my body wasn't itself, wasn't my own. I have a faint memory of walking in the moonlight to the bathroom.

And then it all went dark.

Maybe, Just Maybe

THE NEXT FEW hours live in my mind as a montage, a series of scenes and sensations:

Darkness, then dim light.

Red blood on the bathroom tiles.

Warm blood trickling down my chin.

Knife-twisting pain in my ovaries.

A hand on my waist.

My husband's brown eyes.

Light.

My tingling hands gripping the cold toilet seat.

Vomit.

Numb fingertips.

"Call 911."

Vomit.

Blood in the toilet.

A white robe draped over my shaking body.

Two men standing over me.

Paramedics.

Gauze on my mouth.

Blood-pressure cuff around my arm.

A device clamped over my finger.

Dan's voice. "IVF . . . retrieval . . . medications . . . fainted . . . daughter is sleeping."

A paramedic's voice. "Stitches . . . hospital."

I don't remember getting to the ER, but I remember waiting in triage and being hit with a sudden realization: I wasn't invincible to the ravages of IVF, to its risks. You would think that my early experiences with ovarian hyperstimulation syndrome would have forced me to confront that reality many months before, but it hadn't—at least not like this, not with such brute force. I felt mortal. This wasn't a brush with death, of course. It wasn't dire. I would be fine. I would need eleven stitches to reconnect my split bottom lip, but I would be fine. And yet that moment in the ER felt existential.

What had I done to myself? When would this end? Putting it that way makes it sound like I didn't have a choice. But I did. We did. I wanted to cry, but I was too tired and probably still in some degree of shock. I could tell Dan wanted to cry, too. He was looking at me with such a broken heart. I was fighting a losing battle in the civil war raging inside my body. When would I put down arms? When would *we* put down arms? Concede defeat? Let the universe win?

"I remember looking at you and feeling guilty," Dan reflected years later. "That whole thing happened at a time when you had pulled back a bit from our journey, and I felt like I had pushed you to this place. It was easier to ignore—or at least rationalize—the pain when the wounds were not so visible. But this was the moment it all changed. Blood. Loss of consciousness. Open wound. Tears. It all felt like a wake-up call. I was scared."

When we got home in the early morning hours, Dan went upstairs and promptly cleaned up the evidence. He wiped up the blood, the vomit. He emptied the trash of the blood-soaked gauze. He put the robe in the wash. He got the bed ready for me so I could rest before Sid woke up, none the wiser to what her mom had gone through overnight. My mother-in-law, who had stayed at the house with Sid while she slept, wrapped her arms around me, tears in her eyes. She looked at me with the same look her son had given me in the hospital. "Sweetheart," she said, assessing my wound. The cut was a visual representation of how I felt at this point in the IVF journey: beaten up, torn apart, held together by a thread.

I emailed Dr. Hannam directly to let him know about the fall, the stitches, the ER. I told him I was in bed with sore ovaries, that I hadn't had a bowel movement in four days. I let him know that the lab had called with the fertilization update. Of the seventeen eggs that were extracted, nine were mature. Eight of them had fertilized normally. I signed off with my cell number and said I was around all day if he would like to call. I didn't hear from him personally until two days later, in an email.

"A syncopal episode is awful when the fall is bad," he wrote. "Can you tell me about follow-up? Clearly there was soft tissue trauma, but I hope you are not suffering from concussive symptoms . . . I thought I wrote to you directly with this question but don't see any sent email to that effect. I'm sorry for how isolating or uncaring that felt or may feel now. Our phone calls are never quick and when we speak next it shouldn't be quick again. There is a lot to unpack, especially if embryos are not numerous or not of high quality. Seventeen eggs in itself is considered an ideal response, but in relation to your personal story, like you, I'm worried, and waiting."

Dan's cousin had for months been encouraging us to switch clinics and move our file to Dr. Cliff Librach, the owner and founding doctor of Create Fertility Centre. He had miraculously managed to get her pregnant with both of her children, about ten years prior, after an arduous fertility journey that had failed elsewhere. We booked a consult with Dr. Librach for a Sunday evening, after Sid had gone to bed.

Top of mind for us was Stacey's next, and likely final, transfer. We had gotten the results from our latest retrieval. Of the three embryos we sent for genetic testing, one had come back balanced. We had emailed our team, including Dr. Hannam, four or five times about a potential transfer protocol that included some new medications. The protocol had worked for a friend of ours, whose surrogate had experienced four failed transfers, switched up the protocol and got pregnant on the fifth attempt. We wanted Dr. Hannam's thoughts. We couldn't get a response. Stacey's day one was approaching. And he still hadn't called me to see how I was doing. We finally had a video call booked for an upcoming Friday at 2:15 p.m. and blocked off time in our work schedules. This series of emails sums up our experience toward the end of our time at the clinic:

October 29, 2021, 2:57 p.m.: Hi there—just confirming we're still on for our call with Dr. Hannam? It was scheduled for 2:15. We can wait, but wanted to make sure he was still able to join.

3:16 p.m.: Dr. Hannam—didn't hear back from reception. Just confirming you're still able to make our 2:15 scheduled Zoom?

3:39 p.m.: Haven't heard back from anybody. We are still waiting for our scheduled 2:15 Zoom call with Dr. Hannam. Can someone let us know if he's going to be joining?

5:01 p.m.: We've been waiting for 2 hours and 45 minutes and Dr. Hannam still hasn't showed up for our scheduled Zoom call today. I'm going to assume he isn't that far behind and close the window. We would really like to talk to him—when is he available early next week?

7:36 p.m.: Dear Kathryn Baum, Dr. Hannam informed me to contact you regarding your next frozen embryo transfer (FET) cycle because you are eligible to participate in our research study. If you are thinking about enrolling in an FET within the next few months, we would like to invite you to participate. It is called the CTRA stress study and investigates the topic of stress impacting pregnancy outcomes during FETs. If stress is a factor in pregnancy, we hope to be able to implement stress reduction techniques to improve pregnancy outcomes in the future.

The day of the appointment came and went, and the effort to connect with Dr. Hannam after he missed our appointment continued.

October 31: Following up on the below. Any update? Thanks.

November 1: Hi Kathryn & Dan, I am really sorry you were not able to connect with Dr. Hannam. I will speak with the team and see when we are able to reschedule your appointment.

November 2: Just following up here. Any sense for Dr. Hannam's availability? Haven't heard anything since he missed our scheduled appointment on Friday.

November 3: You are scheduled in for today November 3rd at 11:00 a.m.

We got three hours' notice, on a workday, about the new appointment time. We took the slot and logged on. During the video call, I sat quietly with my fat lip and let Dr. Hannam speak. I don't recall much of what he said, but I do remember he agreed with us that it was probably time to part ways, for us to move on to another clinic that works more often with surrogates, for us to get fresh eyes on our file. Hannam's surrogacy program was small, and it seemed to us that they didn't have the team or infrastructure in place to navigate the intricacies of surrogacy. (In 2022, the clinic suspended its surrogacy program.)

I remember letting Dan do most of the talking, too upset to discuss protocols and plans. At the end of the call, I piped up, my voice shaking. From what I recollect, I told him I couldn't fathom being in his position and not immediately checking in on my patient after such a gory treatment-related injury; that I had expected more from him; that I had felt abandoned at my lowest moment, when I needed him most; that he and his team had made our already punishing journey ever harder with their poor communication, particularly of late.

He looked into the camera and apologized.

"Thank you," I recall saying. "I appreciate that."

I know several people who had seamless and successful journeys at Hannam. They speak highly of their doctors and nursing teams. It's possible they had better experiences because their cases were more straightforward, because they ended up with a baby. It's possible our experience would have been just as hair-pulling elsewhere. It's possible we could have had a frustrating start to our journey at a different clinic and then ended up making a baby at Hannam and leaving the happiest of customers. We will never know. The pandemic didn't help. It caused upheaval across the board, and fertility care was no different. Everyone was doing their best. Dr. Hannam was doing his best.

The truth of the matter, though, is that poor dialogue with clinics is one of the chief complaints among fertility patients. As one woman put it to me about her time at a different clinic, "Communications were God-fucking-awful." Clinics have opened in recent years with the stated goal of improving the patient experience while at the same time providing top-notch medical care, typically at a premium cost.

Some of them use an app to relay lab results, appointment times and medication instructions directly to their patients. That alone could mark a significant improvement in the customer experience, both in terms of transparency and efficiency. Clinics old and new are also increasingly hiring in-house social workers to better support patients. It's a trend I can get behind, though I'm aware that even the best intentions might be met with resistance. Patients seeking medical answers and face time with their doctors may take little comfort in the offer of emotional support.

We decided to transfer our remaining embryos to Create, where we would be patients of Dr. Librach. It was the end of an era. No more emails or calls from or with Hannam. No more taking the elevator to the fifteenth floor. After two years with the clinic and no pregnancy, it was a relief to make the switch. We were under no grand illusion that changing clinics would be the magic bullet, but it was clearly time to move on, if for no other reason than our mental health. A shift in clinics can cause a shift in the mind. We had heard stories of people moving clinics and making babies. Different protocols. Fresh eyes.

Walking into Create on the eleventh floor of a downtown Toronto commercial building, it was apparent the clinic did a ton of volume. The waiting room could accommodate dozens of patients, with row upon row of armchairs facing the main reception desk at the centre of the office. It had an entirely different feel from Hannam—more mom-and-pop, more action, a more tired facility featuring handwritten files stacked on shelves. The walls were tacked with baby photos and thank-you cards.

Doctors, nurses and ultrasound technicians hustled from one room to the next, moving from patient to patient to patient, carrying files and binders, calling out first names and last initials. Everyone seemed to move with a sense of urgency. And yet the clinic was notorious for having its patients wait for hours on end to be seen. You learn to accept the fact that while your appointment is booked for 8 a.m., you might not be through with your clinic visit until the afternoon. That explained the massage chairs at the back of the waiting room, the muted TVs airing the news and the desks and outlets for laptops and phones. Here, we were one of many. And yet we felt more connected to the process than we had in a long time, in part because we could actually *see* the doctors. The white coats were moving around in plain sight, having in-person conversations with their patients. They weren't gatekept by nurses or tucked away in some segregated part of the clinic, only to be seen in the procedure room. It was refreshing. It was what we needed.

Dr. Librach, for his part, has a sort of mad-scientist air about him. On our initial consult call, I thought to myself, "Okay, this guy doesn't have the most traditional bedside manner, but he seems to eat, sleep and breathe fertility." Upon meeting him in person, we found him to be present and reassuring. It felt like he would get shit done, like he would indulge our desire to try some approaches that maybe weren't proven in randomized control trials but had showed promise. I felt like he saw a tough case as an intellectual challenge over which he would triumph. "We want to do things that are based on evidence, but you do have to think outside the box and be more creative," Dr. Librach told me, reflecting on our case years later.

Dr. Librach, who is a professor in the Department of Obstetrics and Gynecology at the University of Toronto, is a fixture in the Canadian fertility community and in the industry more broadly. He started practising in 1991 and founded his clinic less than a decade later. His reputation precedes him, one way or another. There are people who sing his praises, and there are those who deride him as crass and overly aggressive with his treatment. One former patient said he took a phone call on his cell while he was performing her pelvic exam. "It felt vulgar," she said when I let her know we were thinking of switching our care over to him. (I asked Dr. Librach about this years later, and he said he only takes calls when he's with patients if it's regarding a medical issue that requires his immediate attention.) I could understand why the former patient felt put off, but as long as Dr. Librach was kind to Stacey and she was comfortable with him, I was fine with his eccentricities, his juggling act. We knew one day our file would be one of the balls he was trying to keep in the air.

Stacey's first appointment took several hours to get through, on a Saturday no less, but she liked Dr. Librach and felt as though his team was engaged. "I felt more supported," she told me. "He was an oddball, but he was very personable and had good energy . . . You could tell he really cares about what he does. It didn't feel like 'Okay, next.'"

Our Facebook page had by this point garnered a surprising number of responses, but nothing particularly serious or viable had materialized. We were still on the waiting list at a second Canadian surrogacy agency, which we had signed on with more than two years prior, though we had asked them to put our file on pause after we matched with Stacey through CFC. Now that we were potentially looking to be rematched, we were forty-seventh on their list.

We had no idea that working with two agencies was considered taboo, that it was wrong of us to pay two agencies their relatively small initial fee to put us on their respective waitlists. Perhaps this was obvious to some, but we didn't know better. Apparently, we had made a big, big mistake. Unbeknownst to us, the second agency posted our video to their Facebook page, and our contact at CFC saw it. She wrote us an email, cc'ing Leia Swanberg, who was at the time the head of the agency. "There must be a mistake," Swanberg responded. "These intended parents wouldn't be working with another agency. If, in fact, they are, we will need to book a call to discuss next steps."

Dan responded with an email apologizing profusely for our ignorance, tail between his legs. We emailed the second agency and asked them to remove our profile, wanting to make things right with CFC. "I really appreciate the explanation," our CFC contact wrote us. "You are right, it did catch us off guard, and we want to make sure that when we post you on our social media, surrogates don't question why you are shopping at multiple agencies. It also gives them a sense of protection when they know you are committed to one place." Swanberg later told me that when surrogates see the same profiles at multiple agencies, they wonder if the intended parents are getting more than one surrogate pregnant at the same time. She said these days, CFC explicitly communicates to intended parents that it will not work with people who have signed up with multiple agencies.

We felt sick. We had angered the agency at a particularly vulnerable juncture. We needed everyone on our side, rooting for us, helping us move the ball forward. In our effort to optimize and dual track and hedge our bets, had we messed it all up? What was stopping the agency from setting us aside, dragging their feet in rematching us? We had already paid them their sizable consulting fee when we matched with Stacey. They wouldn't be making any more money off us if we needed to be rematched. What was the agency's incentive to include our profile in the pool of intended parents presented to surrogates? If the surrogate matched with a new intended parent, the agency would rake in a new consulting fee. If the surrogate matched with us, the agency would make no additional cash.

Alison Motluk, the journalist who has been covering the fertility beat for many years, has done some digging on this exact scenario. The rematch list, Motluk reported in her 2023 *Hazlitt* piece, is known as "the graveyard" to insiders at CFC. "When new surrogates are recruited, three people who have worked at CFC told me, they are typically first offered to the new clients—known internally as 'money matches' or 'money clients,' because finding surrogates for those people will lead to the payment of a new consulting fee," Motluk wrote. "Sometimes there were explicit instructions in group chat messages to employees to avoid helping people on the rematch list, like one that read, 'Please do not make any more rematches . . .' and another that read, 'We cannot afford rematches at the moment.'"

Motluk's piece went on: "Three people who have worked there say that parents on the rematch list are often just shown profiles of women who are not actually available—they are in the process of being matched to other clients." This gave the intended parents a false sense of hope that they were getting closer to being rematched. Motluk quoted Scott Swanberg, the CEO of the agency and Swanberg's ex-husband, as saying that while he couldn't speak to the past, "we most certainly wouldn't do that now."

I spoke with Leia Swanberg after the *Hazlitt* piece was published. She told me "there's no secret within the agency" that there's a rematch graveyard. "People go there, they get discouraged, they lose hope, they lose steam," she said. She said there are several reasons it can take awhile for those intended parents to be rematched. Sometimes they themselves take a break from the journey. Sometimes surrogates are concerned there's a reason the intended parents had so many failed transfers with their previous surrogate, wondering if there's something amiss with the embryos.

Asked about the lack of financial incentive to get people off the rematch list, Swanberg said the agency is a business and must function as such. Staff must balance the needs of new intended parents with those of intended parents on the rematch list. She also said intended parents needing to be rematched are sometimes charged an administrative fee of several thousand dollars, so she pushed back at the notion that the agency has nothing to gain financially from connecting those people with surrogates. All that being said, Swanberg said it doesn't make sense to leave intended parents in the lurch because of the reputational damage that would do to the agency. "The internet is vicious," she said, alluding to active Facebook groups in the surrogacy space.

In early 2025, Swanberg said CFC hired marketing firms such as Colt's Not My Tummy to help clients get out of the rematch graveyard. (Colt told me that in the first few months of working with CFC-affiliated intended parents, several couples found a rematch by going public with Not My Tummy's support.) As always, Swanberg said, surrogates looking for intended parents have access to the profiles of those who are looking to be rematched. Effectively, she said, they're still in the mix. "We're doing anything we can to keep people moving forward," she said.

In late 2021, with the holiday season upon us, Stacey called in her day one to Create for the first time. The transfer protocol was in place. In addition to the usual suspects of estrogen and progesterone, Dr. Librach's plan included several add-ons, including platelet-rich plasma (PRP) treatment and a couple sessions of intralipid infusion, at a cost of $330 per drip. Reflecting on the treatment plan, Dr. Librach explained that there's good evidence to support PRP in encouraging the uterine lining to become receptive to an embryo seeking to implant. Intralipid infusion, he said, has been shown to improve implantation rates in his clinic, but the basis for its use isn't well-established. The thinking is that an intralipid drip, which is made up of soybean, eggs and peanuts, may calm down natural killer cells and in turn reduce an immune reaction to a transferred embryo, improving the odds of implantation.

Stacey drove back into the city on December 20, 2021, for what we knew would be her final transfer. Afterward, she took a photo with Dr. Librach, his arm around her as she held a sonogram image of her uterus from the moment the embryo was deposited. They were both smiling from ear to ear under their face masks. I saw hope in their eyes, felt it within myself. Maybe this was it. Maybe we had finally done it. Maybe, just maybe, it was our time.

Because of lab closures over the holidays, we were due to get the results from her bloodwork on New Year's Eve while up north at the cottage with Dan's mom, sisters and nieces. Either we would ring in 2022 with a pregnancy, or we would be dealt the final blow of 2021. I woke up on December 31 to a winter wonderland. Sid crawled into bed with us, nestling her head of wispy blond curls under my arm. We went skating on the lake, Sid a little Bambi with her flailing limbs and wobbly knees. I was feeling tired and decided to leave a bit early to return to the cottage. On the walk back, an ache set in. Every joint was overcome with a dull soreness that I recognized as a symptom of the flu. I took my temperature. Fever. I took a rapid COVID test. Positive. Nearly two years into the pandemic, the coronavirus had finally got me. I was looking at two pink lines but not the kind we wanted.

I isolated in our bedroom in the hopes that I could avoid spreading the infection, intermittently sleeping and reading—anything to distract myself from the pending hCG results. We were still waiting on Stacey's bloodwork.

An hour passed.

Then another.

Then another.

And another.

Stacey kept checking an online portal for the bloodwork results, but they weren't yet in.

5:58 p.m. "I'm guessing if nothing by 6, we're probably not hearing tonight?" Dan wrote to Stacey on our group chat.

7:33 p.m. "Anything?" he texted.

8:25 p.m. "I will check now," Stacey responded.

8:29 p.m. "Thanks," Dan wrote.

It was so late that I figured she would tell us there were still no results, but my heart raced nonetheless. I was lying in bed alone, feverish with cold sweats. My body hurt against the mattress. My hips and tailbone felt bruised, as if I had slept on a hardwood floor the night before. Dan was downstairs with Sid. We had let her stay up for an early New Year's Eve countdown. I could hear the family on the main floor chatting. Kids laughing. Cutlery clanging on plates as dishes were cleared from the dining table. The beat of music I couldn't quite make out.

The anticipation was killing me. *Please God or whoever you are or whatever you are, please, please, please don't tell us no. Please, universe, please.*

8:31 p.m. "I'm sorry, guys," Stacey wrote. "I don't know what else to say. I feel like a broken record. My heart hurts for you."

8:32 p.m. "We're sorry," Dan replied. "You are the best."

The bedroom door opened. It was Dan. We looked at each other at a loss, at a distance because I was isolating. We were dejected. Resigned. "Happy fucking New Year," he said. I chuckled and shook my head. Neither of us cried. I remember thinking that must mean something, that we must have turned some kind of corner, that we must have entered new territory where the bad news couldn't hurt us the way it used to.

Dan and I blew each other kisses. I told him to give Sid a hug from me. He let out an exhale, shook his head, closed the door and went back downstairs.

Ten, nine, eight, seven, six, five, four, three, two, one.

Happy New Year.

I had become hardened. Time and disappointment had done a number on me, for better or for worse. I was no longer so exposed, so naked to the elements. Each trauma had formed another link in my armour.

"We're both okay," I wrote to my sister-in-law, Eileen, on New Year's Day. "Good vibes only / fortress of happiness. Basically, I'm numb and that's how I'd like to keep it . . . It has the potential to hurt, but if I just will myself to stay numb, I'm okay. I'm not numb without effort. Not numb by default. It takes conscious doing. Selective, effortful numbness."

"There is something really important about getting to the point where it doesn't hurt," she responded. "Before that point, you're more victim."

She hit the nail on the head. I was through with being a victim.

Around this same time, I was confronted with doses of reality that propelled me further toward acceptance, further from victim. Sid came down with a severe case of croup that required an ambulance to the ER, several doses of epinephrine and near admission to the hospital for respiratory support; a friend had brain surgery for a benign tumour threatening her cerebral function; and a close friend began gruelling treatment for cervical cancer.

Her cancer diagnosis and subsequent hysterectomy, radiation and chemotherapy hit me hard. Illness took her uterus just as she and her husband had been about to start trying for a second child. A couple of years later, after she had beaten cervical cancer and the unrelated breast cancer that came next, she and her husband split up. She's one of my only friends with one child. We felt kinship in that shared experience, particularly because neither of us had chosen it. We talked about what it's like to have one child, about navigating her daughter's questions about it, about the way people don't expect it. "It's like, 'Yeah, I *only* have one child, okay? I got cancer, lost my uterus and got a divorce. Gimme a break,'" she said, incredulous. "Life happened."

I wasn't sick. I didn't have cancer. I had my health. And because of that, I didn't feel so entitled to my sadness anymore. It wasn't that I was denying myself permission to be frustrated that life wasn't going the way I had envisioned. It was that I wasn't taking such advantage of that permission anymore. It wasn't serving me. No amount of tears would get us to Baby in Arms any sooner. It was natural to be sad, of course, but if I could control my emotions—and that was the one thing I *could* control—then I was going forth within a Fortress of Happy. I was choosing to see the good in my life, to be grateful, to be happy. I gave negative feelings and thoughts as little airtime in my mind as was humanly possible. You could call this toxic positivity. You could call it a facade. For me, though, it was pure and true. It was an act of liberation and self-preservation. As much as I was limiting the spectrum of my emotions, restricting myself to good vibes only, I felt freer than I had in a long time.

I knew something had shifted when Sid asked me to wish upon a star with her one evening. "Star light, star bright, first star I see tonight," she said, looking up at the dark sky. "I wish I may, I wish I might, have the wish I wish tonight." For the first time in a long time, I didn't wish for another baby. I wished for our family to be happy, healthy and safe. After all, that *was* what I wanted more than anything. Sid's fourth birthday was approaching, and this time, I would have no mixed emotions.

Years later, I had a fascinating conversation with my friend Tim, who has two children with his husband. It took three women to bring their family into existence—two egg donors and one surrogate. We talked about what made his journey emotionally different from mine and about what might make the gay male experience unique in the realm of IVF. "There's no embarrassment, no shame," he said. "You're just so grateful. It's a feeling of 'I can't believe we get to do this.'" He began his journey firmly rooted in gratitude.

Dan and I had become close with Stacey and her family, investing in each other's lives, so it was emotional to continue our journeys separately—us with another surrogate, and her, potentially, with other intended parents. I think what made our parting of ways easier was that it wasn't abrupt or definite. Time passed, and things became clearer.

When I spoke with Stacey years later about our journey together, I asked her what it was like to have to keep delivering bad news, to have no answers as to why the transfers weren't working, to have to effectively "break up" when there was no discernible reason. She said she felt blindsided each time she got a negative hCG result, as I had earlier in our quest. It was easy for her to get pregnant naturally, so she assumed the first transfer would work, if not the second, third or, for goodness' sake, the fourth. She had taken it as a foregone conclusion; when she left Hannam after a transfer, she thought to herself, "I'm pregnant."

"Because of that, there was a loss in a sense," she told me. "I had such a strong connection with you guys at that point that I wanted it to work so badly. I got the negative pregnancy test and was like, 'How is that even possible?' The thought of breaking that news to you guys was the worst. My stomach was in knots. I just didn't want those words coming out of my mouth. I knew how I felt, and I couldn't imagine what it was like for you guys. You had given me a part of you, and I let that piece go. It was gut-wrenching."

In addition to mentally moving on from doing a journey with Stacey, we probably needed to make more embryos (we had one euploid remaining and one mosaic), and I was reluctant to do another retrieval. I had promised myself that October night in the hospital that I was done. I was scared of ovarian hyperstimulation syndrome. I was scared of fainting again. I was scared of hurting myself in a way that was hard to come back from. After some deliberation and against my better judgment, I decided to do one more retrieval. One more. And that was it. I meant it this time. We wanted to give Dr. Librach a chance at making embryos. Perhaps Create, for one reason or another, would have better luck creating embryos that would actually implant. What would be different about a retrieval at Create? The medications, save for the trigger drugs, would be more or less the same. But the lab and fertilization process, Dr. Librach said, would be different in what he believed to be meaningful ways.

His lab uses technology that functions as an incubator but also takes time-lapsed images of the developing embryos every twenty minutes—without an embryologist removing the embryos from their cozy environment, which is set to a precise temperature and pH level. The device also functions as an embryo-selection tool, using the embryos' cell-division pattern to predict which ones are most likely to implant. He also said the clinic has what he describes as a world-class, in-house genetic-testing lab.

When I started the medications and cycle monitoring, our Facebook page had garnered messages from women who seemed like plausible candidates. Two of them had good support systems and stable jobs and relationships. We could see ourselves getting along and enjoying our time together, separate from the task at hand. We scheduled video calls with both of them. One woman, Nicole, told us that she had gone down the road of potentially being a surrogate back in 2019, but the pandemic interrupted her journey with a couple living abroad, which never came to fruition. She seemed lovely. The other, Kendra, thirty-nine, was married with three children and lived in a rural area about an hour-and-a-half drive outside the city. We pretty quickly realized they lived on a property along the route we take to the cottage; we'd driven by their home more times than we could count.

Kendra and her husband, Sebastien, appeared on our screen, and I immediately felt drawn to them. The more we spoke, the more comfortable I felt. I remember taking Dan's hand and squeezing it, as if to say "I like them. Do you?" We talked about where we were in our journey and about why Kendra was interested in being a surrogate. She told us it broke her heart to think of people wanting a baby but not being able to have that experience, for one reason or another. She knew the joy of having children, and if she could help someone start or grow their family, she was open to the possibility of helping. She hadn't been actively looking to do a surrogacy journey. She wasn't signed up with an agency. She had seen our post while scrolling Facebook and was intrigued.

As part of my reporting for this book, I asked Kendra what it was about us that stood out to her. She's a bit shy so she asked if she could provide her responses to my questions in writing. It turned out to be the best approach, since some of her answers were inevitably quite personal and likely to stir emotions in one or both of us. "At the time I stumbled across the Facebook post, I was at a point in my life where I was seeking more purpose," she wrote. "I guess I felt as though I wanted to accomplish something more and didn't feel entirely fulfilled . . . I saw the photo of you guys and Sid and was intrigued as to why you were needing a surrogate when you clearly had a child already. It made me want to read your story, and you seemed like such a nice family. I knew after each child I'd had that I didn't feel quite complete yet, so I totally understood your desire to give Sid a sibling and grow your family."

On our first video call, we laughed about how strange it was to meet someone online and discuss making a baby together. Their three kids entered the frame, one of them wearing a silly winter hat with long ears that could be tied under the chin. "You're such a goof," Kendra said. The kids laughed, and so did we. From our perspective, our "first date" had gone well. We hoped they felt the same. And they did. Kendra had been nervous to meet us, but she felt a sense of calmness come over her within a few minutes of speaking. Seb, for his part, was initially apprehensive about the idea of Kendra becoming a surrogate because of the implications it could have for their family. They were both working full-time and raising three kids, so life was busy and stressful enough. Ultimately, though, he was on board with supporting her through a journey he knew was important to her.

CFC told us we should introduce any potentially viable candidates to them for screening. We had second video calls with both Nicole and Kendra so they could better get to know us and so we could decide whom we would like to proceed with. Again, this was taboo and we had no idea. We didn't know CFC would view it as distasteful that we were speaking with two women at once, despite having found them ourselves through Facebook. We were transparent with both of them that we were chatting with other women, but apparently, by Swanberg's standards, we were very much in the wrong. She called us, irate. We were leading these women on. Didn't we know how offside this was? Speaking to two potential surrogates at the same time was messy. If they found out about each other, they might think we were trying to get two women pregnant so that we could embark on a sneaky tandem journey. And while we were clear we weren't necessarily moving forward with them, they might be forgoing discussions with other prospective intended parents and could lose the opportunity to carry for another worthy couple.

Ms. Swanberg all but threatened to drop us as clients. She said she had called Dr. Librach to ask his opinion of Dan and me, and "for some reason" he had "vouched" for us and said we were "good people." I swore to her that we were, indeed, good people. Years later, Ms. Swanberg explained to me that she called Dr. Librach because he knows his patients and she wanted to hear his opinion of us; she said she feels it's important to have a direct line of communication to people like Dr. Librach, for example, in the case of a medical emergency involving a CFC surrogate receiving treatment at his clinic.

Dan did his best to do damage control. I sobbed at the thought that we had done something wrong, that we might be punished for it. I was hormonal, my estrogen through the roof from the retrieval meds. I don't remember where we were coming from when the call came in, but when it ended, we were in our driveway. It was raining. I was so totally overwhelmed. I curled up in the car's front seat and kept crying, my pants bursting at the button with the pressure from my bloated stomach. How much could one person take?

I asked Ms. Swanberg about this interaction in one of the conversations we had years later. She reiterated that she had been too hard on intended parents in the past, but she was also firm in her belief that continuing to speak with both women at once would have ended poorly. "The way I delivered the news, again, had an impact on you," she said. "And also, had you continued talking to them, you would have lost them both."

The second time I woke up on the bathroom floor in the middle of the night, there was no blood. This time when I fainted, Dan had caught me and lowered me to the ground. I had just done a pre-retrieval trigger injection, which had to be done around 2 a.m. the day before the extraction. Given what had happened the last time I was on medications and got up in the middle of the night, Dan insisted on coming with me to the bathroom for the injection.

Next thing I knew, I was on the floor, fluttering open my eyes. Again. "What happened?" I cried, shaking and confused. "You fainted," he said. My hands went tingly and then numb. Again. I proceeded to vomit with such violence that I broke blood vessels in my eyes. It was as if I was having labour contractions, but instead of delivering a baby, I was spewing bile from my efforts to make one. Something felt very much the matter. "I think you need to call 911," I managed to utter.

The paramedics arrived and helped me off the bathroom floor and into our bed. I could not stop puking. I could barely lift my head to aim for a garbage pail, so they gave me a bunch of disposable vomit bags that I could hold under my mouth and then pass along when it got full. The abdominal spasms were so forceful that I wet the bed. Tears streaming down my face, I begged for it to be over.

The paramedics said that though I'd had another fainting spell and I was still vomiting, I was safe to stay home and didn't need to go to the hospital. By now it was about 3:30 a.m. I called an emergency number I had for Dr. Librach. I wanted to make sure he wasn't overly worried about what was happening, that he was comfortable with me not going to ER. I was concerned my ovaries might burst or something gnarly, and I needed to hear from my doctor that I was okay. Dr. Librach called me right back. He was kind and reassuring. He explained that my blood pressure had probably been a bit out of whack and I had likely gone into shock, hence the tingling hands, nausea and vomiting. As long as things didn't get worse, I could ride it out at home. If I got dehydrated from all the puking, I should go into the clinic for an IV drip. The paramedics stayed until my vitals were closer to my norm and then went on their way.

The puking went on for a couple more hours. I was dizzy from how bad the nausea was. Dan was kneeling beside me, holding whatever part of my body wasn't writhing. He had tears in his eyes. "I can't do this anymore," I told him, my throat burning from the acid. "You can't let me. After this retrieval, I have to be done. You have to make me be done."

"Okay," he said. "I know. I will. You're done."

He sat with me until I eventually fell asleep, around the time Sid woke up to start her day. Mama isn't feeling well, Dan told her. Dada would be taking her to daycare today. I texted my editor to let him know what had happened. "Had quite the night," I said and then described in broad strokes what transpired. "Anyhow, I got some writing done on the health-care story over the weekend. I'm hoping I can take it across the finish line today, from bed. Because tomorrow is a write-off (I'll be sedated etc. for the retrieval) . . . And by the way, I'm done with IVF treatments. I can't endure any more. I'll be back in more consistent fighting strength soon."

"Oh god," he wrote back. "So sorry to hear this. You have been through so much—you and your family. It's unfathomable, really, how strong you've been. I hope this decision brings you some closure on one chapter." A story was due, and he made no mention of it. I was so fortunate to work with people who welcomed transparency and showed compassion.

On retrieval day, Dr. Librach harvested fifty-two eggs. Of those, thirty-four were mature and twenty-seven had fertilized normally. That's a massive number. And despite the volume, I wasn't suffering from ovarian hyperstimulation syndrome. (I spoke with a woman who was also treated by Dr. Librach; she said she experienced OHSS on two of her retrieval cycles, in which she said around forty eggs were extracted each time, and she had to have fluid drained on both occasions.)

I wondered if I didn't get OHSS because I wasn't triggered with hCG. Praise be. Things were looking up. And regardless, I was done. It was over for me, even if our journey wasn't. Over and out.

The Man

I DOVE INTO the pool at Toronto Metropolitan University and felt the cool water subsume my body. It had been twenty-five years since I had put on a swim cap, spat in my goggles and rubbed the lenses to keep them from fogging up. The last time I had done drills with a coach, I was a kid. I felt like one again, for the first time in forever. The smell of chlorine, the goosebumps before I was warmed up, the black marker on the whiteboard outlining the plan for the session. Pull. Kick. Free. Fins. Breathwork. Ascending. Descending. Build. Cool down. It was all so familiar.

It was 6 a.m. on a rainy spring morning, and there was nowhere else I wanted to be. The pool—specifically in a lane—is my happy place. I had forgotten that. When I was officially done giving my body over to fertility treatment, I decided to fully reclaim it. I decided to celebrate it, cherish it, enjoy it. I had always been a runner. I had a few years prior gotten into cycling. I was a competitive swimmer as a child. What was stopping me from becoming a triathlete? Finally, nothing. I signed up for a race in Ontario that upcoming summer, found a swim group to train with and printed off a training schedule.

A perk of having one kid was the time to do something like this. I took advantage.

We were in a good place. The fifth and final retrieval—our only one at Create—had gleaned two balanced embryos and one low mosaic. The conversion from the number of mature eggs retrieved to fertilized was quite poor, but the outcome itself was decent. We now had three balanced embryos and two low mosaics. We had two lovely women who were willing to do a surrogacy journey with us, and we were in the enviable position of deciding between them. We chose to proceed with Kendra. Our Facebook exchanges and conversations with her were easy, flowing. She seemed trustworthy and kind, and her husband was supportive and had a good sense of humour. She passed the medical and psychological screening, and we signed a legal contract and got her set up with life insurance. We were much more adept at this whole "intended parent thing" by now. We felt more comfortable, which I think helped Kendra feel more at ease too.

I joined Kendra at her medication teaching session at Create, where a nurse showed her how and where to inject the drugs. I had no idea she had a needle phobia. She knew she would have to do some injections, but it wasn't until she was in the room with the syringes that she realized what exactly she had signed up for. She nearly fainted when the nurse showed her the needle she would be using. Her face drained of colour, and she looked terrified. I, too, was terrified. I was nervous she would back out. But Kendra isn't a quitter. She has a tattoo of the acronym H.O.P.E.—"hold on, pain ends"—on her ankle. Fear wasn't going to stop her from fulfilling a dream she'd had for several years, from fulfilling our dream. Her husband would help with the injections. The nurse and I promised her it would get easier with time.

After the appointment, our families met up at the Ontario Science Centre so we could meet each other's kids and have an afternoon together. Kendra's kids, aged eight, eleven and thirteen at the time, were enamoured with Sid. They thought she was adorable, walking through the lily-pad installation, dropping marbles through a kinetic maze, giggling at her reflection in fun-house mirrors, fishing for plastic toys in the water-play area. At one point, Kendra's eldest daughter, a naturally gifted artist, picked up a pencil and a piece of paper and sketched an image of Sid. The likeness was impressive. The gesture was heartwarming. I kept the drawing and tucked it into Sid's keepsake box, hoping it would hold significant meaning one day, a point to plot.

Kendra's transfer protocol was similar to what Dr. Librach had tried with Stacey. On April 29, 2022, I sat with Kendra in the procedure waiting area for what felt like hours. Wearing hair covers and blue gowns, we took a selfie together, our fingers crossed. "I love this woman," I texted Dan, who was sitting in the main waiting area, trying to tame his anxiety by creating a list of questions for us to ask Dr. Librach after the transfer. "She's so easy to talk to. Really sweet."

About two hours later than scheduled, we were called into the procedure room. I sat by Kendra's head, my hand on her shoulder. We were adults, both women, and she was about to try to get knocked up with my baby, but it was still awkward being in such close proximity when her feet were in stirrups. "hCG espresso shots are in," I updated Dan by text, referring to the injection of hCG into the uterus prior to a transfer. Dr. Librach had likened it to a shot of espresso, helping to kickstart the embryo's growth. "Librach said the uterus looks beautiful. Kendra says to cheer on Baby Baum No. 2."

I laced up my runners and made my way to the starting line of an annual ten-kilometre race through the city. It was Mother's Day, nine days post-transfer, and I was looking forward to losing myself in the runner's high. We had decided with Kendra that she wouldn't test until after the weekend, as we both wanted to spend time with our families without the prospect of bad news. She would pee on a stick with her first urine on Monday morning and then message us with the result. That way, if it was negative, we would all have a minute to gather ourselves before speaking on the phone after the kids left for school.

Off I went that Sunday morning, singing along to my running mix, Sigrid's "Don't Kill My Vibe" blasting in my earbuds. I'm sure the song has a specific meaning to the artist, but when I listened, it was about my relationship with suffering. Pain, I was okay with. Suffering, go fuck yourself. *You think you're so important to me, don't you? You don't belong here. Don't kill my vibe.*

I was wearing my new Apple watch, which I had bought to track my training for the upcoming triathlon. It started lighting up with messages. A couple of days prior, Kendra had tested positive for COVID. She had a cough, sore throat and a headache but no fever, aches or trouble breathing. We were doing our best to remain calm and not spiral. We were concerned for Kendra's health, of course. COVID is an odd beast. You never know who would get hit hard and who would have mild symptoms. We were also concerned about what this meant for a potential pregnancy. We figured it wasn't ideal for implantation. When Kendra texted saying her symptoms had ramped up and her chest felt heavy, my stomach dropped. She decided to go to the hospital to be safe.

I was running down Yonge Street when the next text came in. The doctor said Kendra's lungs sounded good and that she needed to let her body fight off the infection. He also suggested she do bloodwork then and there to determine whether she was pregnant. That way, she wouldn't have to make a separate trip to a lab the following day while feeling so unwell. It would be about an hour till we would get the results. My heart rate picked up as I continued to run.

I was in my head when I saw a runner in front of me gaze up at a high-rise condo building. I looked to see what was so interesting but didn't notice anything. I looked again at the man, who was now sort of running backward, flailing, looking at the sky, trying not to stumble. And then his body gave out and he hit the ground, his head bouncing off the concrete. He had fainted. He was unconscious, not moving. Runners ran by, continuing with their race, either oblivious or choosing not to get involved in whatever was happening. I sprinted over and knelt beside him, yanking out my headphones and calling out for a doctor. A woman ran over. She untied a jacket from around her waist and tucked it under the man's head. Someone called 911. The man, who appeared to be in his twenties, started seizing, foaming at the mouth. His body went rigid, his eyes bulged, his lips turned blue. I thought I was watching him die. I kept saying to him, "You're okay. It's okay. You're okay. It's okay. We're here. You're okay." I had a flashback to when Dan had assured me the same when I woke up on the bathroom floor.

The paramedics arrived and took over. The man regained consciousness, and the colour started coming back to his face. The paramedics put him on a stretcher and loaded him into an ambulance. I never found out what happened to him, but the doctor who had helped tend to him assured me he would be okay. I sat on the curb for a few minutes, a stampede of feet pounding the pavement in front of me. I was rattled. After taking a few minutes to gather myself, I rejoined the mass of joggers and finished the race.

Dan and Sid would have normally met me there, but they were at an arcade with my nephew. I jogged home from the race, figuring I may as well get in the extra training kilometres. When I got home, I hopped in the shower, praying for some Mother's Day good news. How perfect would that be?

Dan was still out with Sid when Kendra's text came through with the results. The first thing I saw was a sad-face emoji. Then some of the words jumped out to me: *So sorry. Didn't work. Disappointed.* I called Dan and asked if he had seen the message. He had. Neither of us cried. I didn't have to pretend to be okay. I *was* okay. Maybe not as chipper as I sounded in my response to Kendra, but better than any other time we'd gotten negative results. We knew she would be gutted, and we didn't want to pile on. It was important that we support her.

"Awww not the news we wanted but we gotta keep our chins up!" I wrote. "First priority now is for you to get better. Darn COVID. Lots of love."

"Was driving home through tears," she responded. "This is harder than I thought. I keep going over the reasons why it wouldn't work in my head, and I just don't understand . . . I'm not having an easy time with this, so I can't imagine you two."

"It's not easy, but there's nothing you did that made it not work," Dan chimed in. "And as the doctor said, your uterus is perfect. Sometimes it just doesn't work. This is the hardest part. Tomorrow will be a little bit easier. And the next one will be the one! We got this. Wish we could give you a big hug."

There was no obvious reason the transfer hadn't worked. For Kendra, the news hit her almost as hard as it would have if it had been in pursuit of her own child. And while she was dreading going through another round of medications, she was ready to try again when she got her next period. "Go team Baby Baum!" she wrote, feeling more optimistic. "I'm staying strong and positive."

A couple of days later, we got a message from Stacey. She had been wanting to find a time to chat and check in on us. And to tell us something. "We are pregnant," her text said. "This is probably the hardest thing I've had to tell you guys and I've really been struggling with it . . . I feel like I'm throwing salt in your wound. We went through so much, and it feels like a slap in the face. I don't have any other words to say how sorry I am that this didn't work out between us. I really do wish you guys all the best and understand if this is just too hard for you and have to cut all ties."

I was in the newsroom on deadline when the text came in, working on a quick-turnaround story about the federal government's climate-change adaptation strategy. I was surprised she was pregnant, but because it was a natural conception, the news didn't sting in quite the way it would have if she had become pregnant for another couple.

"First of all, congratulations!" I wrote. "This is beautiful news for your family. We're happy for you. Truly, truly. And we will never cut ties with you! You're stuck with us forever, as one of our angels and friends. As for us, we have found another surrogate but no good news to share. Here's to hoping we have a successful transfer sometime soon!"

When Stacey shared that she had been struggling with her pregnancy, I had figured she meant that she felt guilty getting pregnant for herself when she couldn't get pregnant for us. But when I spoke with her years later, I realized it ran much deeper than that. I realized just how invested she had become in our life, our journey, our story. "My attachment to the pregnancy at the beginning was so different from the boys," she shared, referring to her two sons. "I just kept thinking, 'This shouldn't be mine. This should be Kathryn and Dan's.' It was a constant battle within myself. I knew it was genetically mine, but it felt like it was supposed to be yours. I remember thinking, 'Why did this happen?'"

At the time Stacey's text came in, we had Kendra's next transfer to look forward to, to hang our hopes on. This would be our eighth transfer of a genetically balanced embryo. Our second attempt in our third womb. Kendra called in her day one and began the transfer protocol. Her tummy was covered in bruises at various stages of healing, some dark blue, some yellowy, some greenish. Another body taking a beating on my behalf.

One Saturday at the end of May, Kendra met with a nurse at Create for her intralipid infusion. I knew it would be a long day at the clinic, so I brought her some lunch and sat with her, chatting to pass the time as the IV bag dripped, dripped, dripped. It looked like melted vanilla ice cream. Her lining check went well. Her endometrium, again, looked lush. We were on track for a transfer in early June. She was booked for a 7 a.m. transfer, which meant getting up around 4 a.m. to make the drive.

Kendra and her husband got to the clinic early that day and sent us a photo of the two of them in their blue hair covers and gowns. They waited. "So frustrating," Kendra wrote. "No doc yet. I didn't expect that. Not sure why they say 7 and the doctor shows up much later." And waited. "Why would a doc say 7 and it's almost 9 and he's not in? I just don't get that." And waited some more. "I know you can't control it, but it surely blows my mind how they disregard other people's time. Just venting, but it's okay. I'm fine. He will get here eventually and it will get done."

The transfer was done at 9:30 a.m. On the way home, Kendra reclined her seat and relaxed, letting the embryo "get comfy," as she put it. "I'm currently rubbing my belly and saying, 'Come on little embryo, do your thing for your mommy and daddy,'" she wrote to us on the drive home. "Seb is laughing at me, but I figure if I rub my belly with loving vibes, it will want to stay."

Stay, little one, stay.

I was gearing up for a feature to be published on the front page of *The Globe*'s Saturday edition, busy with edits, fact-checking and finalizing visuals with the photo desk and graphics team. The piece was about the impact of rising global temperatures on human health, about how extreme heat is a silent and prolific killer with the power to overwhelm emergency medical services. Work was again a good distraction during the post-transfer wait. And besides, I had put less pressure on this transfer than I ever had. That's just what time had done to me.

We had a busy weekend ahead, with synagogue services and evening celebrations to mark two bat mitzvahs in Dan's family. It was a beautiful Friday night for a backyard party. The sun was shining, and there was a light breeze. No threat of rain. Sid, wearing her favourite peach tutu dress and a silver tiara, was living her best life. Dan and I were glued to each other's side, trying to be present and relish in Sid's joy. We watched as she danced to the Black Eyed Peas' "I Gotta Feeling," her tiara tilted on her head, her cheeks rosy.

And then my phone lit up with a photo of a pregnancy test.

YES+.

"I can't hold it in!" Kendra wrote. "It's too hard. Now go do a happy dance." I grabbed Dan by the arm and rushed him to a corner of the back patio, away from the packed dance floor. I showed him the picture on my phone. "Oh my God," he said. He looked up and we locked eyes. "Oh my God," he said again, looking at the photo once more to make sure his eyes weren't playing tricks. "Let's go out front," I said, taking him by the hand and leading him through the house. We weren't ready for anyone to know anything yet. We went out the front door and around the corner to a side street. I dropped down to a squat and put my head in my hands, crying happy tears. "Is this real?" I said, looking up at Dan. "Is this really real?" I stood up and threw my arms around his neck. We held each other tight. I could feel his body vibrating against mine, this time with relief and disbelief. I pulled back just enough to give him a kiss, and then I wiped his tears. He walked a few paces away, his hands running through his hair as he looked up at the blue sky, in total disbelief. After all we had been through—after so many failed attempts—it was unbelievable, in the truest sense of the word.

"It's so early, but this is major," I remember saying to Dan. "Obviously I don't want to put this into the universe, but no matter what happens, we now know that it's possible for someone to get pregnant with one of our embryos." It was a massive milestone. We both lost our breath, the adrenalin and euphoria taking over. I bent forward and put my hands on my knees, letting out an exhale. "Is this real?" I looked up and asked Dan again. I don't recall who called who, but we ended up on FaceTime with Kendra and her youngest daughter. "It's real, guys," she assured us. "I'm pregnant. You're having a baby!"

"Thank you," I sobbed. "Thank you, thank you. You're an angel."

We knew we didn't want to tell anyone at the party, apart from Dan's mom, who had seen us rush off and was on edge wondering what was going on. Dan took her aside in the backyard and discreetly told her the news. She teared up as she held his face in her hands. She kissed his cheek, used her thumb to wipe her lipstick from his face.

"Thank you, God," she said. "Thank you."

We went over to the dance floor and joined hands with Sid. We danced under the sinking sun, our secret nestled in Kendra's womb. Time slowed. Our spirits soared. After a couple songs, Dan and I went to the bar to get a drink to toast the news. The white wine hit my lips, and I realized then and there how different this would be, already was: We were pregnant, and I was celebrating with a drink.

Is this what it's like to be the man?

So much starts happening inside a person the minute an embryo implants in the uterus—increased blood flow, rising hormones, anatomical changes. But unlike the five pregnancies we'd had till this point, this one wasn't happening in *my* body. We were pregnant, but my body was none the wiser. And while there's something comforting about feeling the proof of pregnancy within yourself, there was also something entirely liberating about feeling nothing at all. I couldn't read into every slight cramp, every bit of nausea or fatigue. I didn't tense up and pray every time I went to the bathroom, felt something in my underwear. I didn't worry that I was bleeding or about to bleed. I competed in my first triathlon and then my second, not worried that I was overdoing it. I dreamed of baby names as I cycled. The disconnect was at once disconcerting and wonderful. Our baby was growing in another garden. The seed was ours, but the soil was not. It was richer.

It's true that cisgender men don't get to experience the miracle of pregnancy—and for all its aches, pains and disruption, it truly is a miracle. But they also don't have to experience what it's like for their body to be taken over by another being, to be consumed, invaded. And while this was as close as I would get to having the male experience of pregnancy, it wasn't perfectly akin. A third person was involved. Because I knew first-hand what it's like to be pregnant, I felt guilty that I was feeling physically myself and Kendra wasn't. I felt personally responsible for her fatigue, her headaches, her aversions.

It was one thing to have outsourced fertility treatment. It was quite another, I was realizing, to outsource the actual pregnancy. There was new life in the mix. It was no longer an intellectual exercise or a hypothetical. I didn't mourn the fact that I wasn't carrying the baby in the way others might, had they never carried before or had they had less of a slog reaching this point. I was so focused on the goal of a baby in arms that I had become agnostic about the location of the womb. And I had more faith in the ability of Kendra's body to bring our baby earthside than I did my own. That's a powerful protective mechanism against negative emotions.

There was no jealousy or insecurity, or at least none that I was conscious of. I wouldn't have judged myself if there had been. It's not natural to watch someone else grow your baby. But if there's enough desperation, trust and gratitude, it can *feel* natural. What was it like for Kendra to be pregnant for someone else? The concept was strange, she reflected, but she knew the baby wasn't hers and was able to stay in that mindset. As with her pregnancies for her own children, she wanted to protect the baby and keep it safe.

I wondered if my feelings about someone else carrying my baby might change at our first ultrasound, when things would become more real. The first scan was scheduled for July 4, 2022—our wedding anniversary and the day before my thirty-eighth birthday. Kendra would be about seven weeks by then. Leading up to the scan, every hour that passed without bad news felt like a gift.

I hadn't even thought about a due date. I hadn't allowed myself to. But Kendra was optimistic and excited, so she used an online calculator to determine that the baby was expected February 20, 2023. She created a profile for the baby on a pregnancy app, tracking the embryo's growth starting from a "sweet pea" at six weeks. "I'm giving people at work goosebumps," she said. "Everyone is so happy for you guys and they have no idea who you are." It was beautiful to think of these complete strangers rooting for us. I was emotional at the thought and joked to Kendra that perhaps her hormones were making me hormonal through osmosis.

We didn't wait till the ultrasound to tell a few of our loved ones, including my close friend and my sister, who had just found out she was pregnant with her third child. If Kendra miscarried, we would want their support anyhow. We weren't as married to secrecy as we had been in pregnancies past. Our sweet pea had grown into a blueberry by the time we had our first ultrasound. The three of us sat in the Create waiting room, chatting while we waited for Kendra's name to be called. It was our turn. Kendra went to the imaging room first to get into her gown and onto the table. When it was time for us to join her, my knees almost buckled as I walked down the hallway. "Please let there be a heartbeat," I said to Dan. He held my clammy hand and knocked on the door.

Anyone who has experienced a loss can relate to the anxiety we felt in that moment. I took Kendra's hand in mine and looked at the monitor, waiting for things to come into focus. And then we saw it. Inside a black sac, there was a grey blob. And inside the grey blob, there was a heart beating, a pulse flickering at a healthy 142 beats per minute. The baby was measuring seven weeks plus one day, right where it should be. I broke out in tears of relief and rested my face on the pillow tucked under Kendra's head. "Thank you," I whispered. To her. To Dr. Librach. To the universe.

Dr. Librach wasn't in that day to review the results, so we met with another doctor whose bedside manner left much to be desired. She told us that the ultrasound picked up a subchorionic hematoma, or SCH, which is effectively a blood clot between the placenta and the uterine wall. This kind of hematoma most commonly arises between ten and twenty weeks of gestation, and they account for somewhere in the order of 10 percent of all vaginal bleeding during pregnancy. They're more common in women with uterine irregularities, those who have a history of miscarriage, those with high blood pressure and, interestingly, those who become pregnant through IVF. I wonder, though, whether hematomas actually happen more frequently in women who do IVF or if those women are more closely monitored and in turn more likely to be diagnosed with an SCH that would have otherwise gone undetected. It's certainly true that women who undergo IVF receive more information than their average counterpart who conceived naturally. That creates more opportunity for (sometimes unnecessary) worry.

Most of the time, a hematoma is benign and resolves on its own without issue, either through a small amount of harmless bleeding or by being reabsorbed by the body. But depending on the size of the SCH and the stage of pregnancy, it can be associated with complications such as excessive bleeding, miscarriage and placental abruption, in which the placenta detaches from the uterus. We were relieved there was a heartbeat, but we were scared that this hematoma would suck the life out of our baby. The doctor, while reassuring, was quite dismissive of our questions, which spoke to the fact that she didn't fully appreciate how long we had fought to get to this point. It was a small hematoma, but it was a big deal to us.

A couple of days later, our nurse was in touch by email, saying that Dr. Librach would monitor the hematoma. "Generally, the clot will expel on its own (and if it does, don't worry) or it can remain throughout pregnancy," she wrote. "It's important to avoid strenuous activity and heavy lifting / strong manoeuvres like vomiting / coughing." We paid for a cleaner to go to Kendra's house once a week so that she wouldn't have to vacuum or mop or use the stairs too much, but how could we reasonably expect her to avoid vomiting if she felt nauseous or prevent coughing if she fell ill?

One thing we did to help alleviate our stress around this time was order Kendra a Doppler, a device that can detect the sound of a fetal heartbeat. We were at the cottage getting ready for bed one night when Kendra sent a video of her using the Doppler. I savoured the sound of our baby's heartbeat. The submersed gallop, the proof of life.

As much as we needed to hear our baby, we also wanted our baby to hear us. We sent Kendra voice notes to play over her belly, sometimes loving words, sometimes a lullaby I tried to sing on key. Kendra had the sweet idea of having stuffed animals made for Sid and the baby. One a deer, the other a moose. Inside their paws, she planned to insert voice recorders with messages from Dan and me. She wanted our kids—especially our baby—to always be able to hear our voices, to always know we were there.

—

Kendra's reassurance—the Doppler reports, the pics of her growing belly, her messages—carried us from one appointment to the next. Had I been the one with the subchorionic hematoma, the anxiety would have been crippling. Not only was Kendra's soil richer, her garden was more tranquil.

We wanted to keep Kendra's stress levels low, so we ordered her some prepared foods to make dinnertime easier. We made sure the cleaner was there once a week. If Kendra had questions about how to file her expenses, we would reach out to the surrogacy agency or check our agreement. We invited her family up to the cottage, about a forty-five-minute drive from their home, to spend time together. The family came for a swim, some fishing and a barbecue dinner. Sid still didn't know Kendra was pregnant with her sibling. To her, the family was simply friends of ours. She bonded especially with Kendra's youngest daughter, who was six years older than Sid—about the same age gap that would exist between Sid and her brother or sister if things went well. It was comforting to see them engage so seamlessly.

Would it be a brother or a sister? We had never been the couple willing to wait until the delivery to find out the sex. This time would be no different. There are scientific methods of determining the baby's sex, including through pre-implantation genetic testing during IVF. In Canada, though, it's illegal for patients to know the sex of an embryo before implantation, except for cases involving sex-linked disorders or diseases. This is to reduce the possibility of sex-selective abortion, which tends to affect female fetuses due to cultural norms that value males.

In the United States, by comparison, IVF patients can not only know whether they made male or female embryos, they can choose which sex to implant. They can choose the makeup of their family. This could be viewed as empowering or burdensome—almost *too* much responsibility. I spoke about this with a Canadian woman who went to Arizona for a transfer of an embryo created with a donor egg and her husband's sperm.

They had been deliberate about selecting their egg donor—it was important to them that the woman be educated and financially stable, that she was informed about the process and not doing it for money. (Egg donors can be compensated in the United States.) They didn't care about hair or eye colour, since their first daughter, who was conceived naturally, has blond hair and blue eyes and they both have brown hair and brown eyes. Such features wouldn't be conspicuous or revealing. It was, however, important to them that the donor be of the same ethnicity as them and have a similar body type. They were thinking ahead and wanted to guard against the child feeling othered from the rest of the family by so clearly standing out. They also wanted an open arrangement as opposed to an anonymous donor, in the event that their future child wanted to contact the donor.

When it came time to choose the sex of the embryo to transfer, the couple was similarly thoughtful, the woman told me. She already had a daughter, so she "already knew how to do that," she said. Her husband wasn't hung up on having a son. In fact, he was happy to have two girls. In addition, she wasn't sure what it would be like to have a child conceived via an egg donor, so she figured it was best to keep variables at bay and stick with what she knew. They chose to transfer a female embryo. She said she felt less attached to the pregnancy than she had with her first-born, but it's unclear to her whether that was a function of the donor element or, more likely, the fact that it was her ninth pregnancy and she had gotten used to protecting her heart. She gave birth in late 2024 to a healthy girl.

On August 8, 2022, when Kendra was about twelve weeks, we went to the clinic for an ultrasound to check on the size of the hematoma, screen for genetic issues and find out the sex. Kendra had done non-invasive prenatal screening, known as NIPT, which looks for certain chromosome abnormalities and can, if the parents wish, reveal the sex of the baby. Because our embryos had been genetically tested before implantation, there had been no good reason for us to do NIPT. The screening effectively does the same thing in utero that pre-implantation genetic testing does in the lab. And yet for peace of mind, we opted to pay the $500 and have the NIPT done to doubly confirm there were no chromosomal abnormalities.

People often say they don't care whether they have a boy or a girl so long as the baby is healthy. Sometimes that's just something people say. In our case, it was the God's honest truth. In years past, Dan had said he would love to have a son, but by this point, all he cared about was that the baby was growing and that the hematoma was not. Nonetheless, we were curious to learn what Kendra was carrying. It would help us better connect with the pregnancy, especially since it was happening outside our home, outside our day-to-day. I have heard men say that they want to know the sex before the delivery because it helps them bond with the unborn baby, picture their life with the child. I understood that sentiment more than ever.

Kendra was called in for the ultrasound, which showed that the pregnancy was developing normally and that the hematoma was gone. It had disappeared. The baby was moving around in Kendra's womb, seemingly waving at us. I kept a sonogram from that ultrasound, our baby's tiny vertebrae and little limbs discernible. We were in such disbelief that things were going so well that we made Dr. Librach repeat the findings.

We had decided Kendra would be the one to reveal the sex to us by giving us a box containing either a floral or grey onesie. Dan and I waited for her outside the clinic on a stoop in the sunshine. Kendra emerged from the building and, with a huge grin on her face, handed us the white box. "Let's see if it's a boy or a girl," she said. I opened the box, slowly peeled back the tissue paper and pulled out the onesie.

Grey.

We were having a boy.

At this point, we had officially graduated from the care of the fertility clinic and needed to find an obstetrician. We had considered getting an OB in Toronto, given that it's the only place we'd had experience with prenatal care and delivery. It was familiar, so it was comfortable. Kendra, for her part, was squeamish about delivering at the regional hospital close to where she lived, after her mother had a less-than-optimal experience with a surgery there. We knew she would need a C-section, given that she'd had C-sections with her own children.

It's uncommon to have a vaginal birth after a C-section, especially after more than two prior C-sections. This is due to the risk of uterine rupture, which occurs when an old C-section scar tears open during labour. While rare, it can be fatal to the patient and the baby.

If we wanted her to deliver in Toronto, she would need an OB in Toronto, which meant all of her appointments would be in the city. None of us liked the thought of Kendra driving an hour and a half on a snowy highway to the city for an appointment in the dead of winter. We agreed it made sense for her to see a local OB, who came highly recommended by Dr. Librach.

Our first appointment with the OB was in early September, when Kendra was about fourteen weeks. It wasn't a major milestone visit, but Dan and I wanted to be there to meet the doctor and be with Kendra. The OB and her staff treated the three of us as if we were typical patients, not some cumbersome, anxious trio. At the initial visit, the OB used a Doppler to check the baby's heart rate. I made a recording, planning to hopefully someday make Kendra a short video capturing her surrogacy journey.

I closed my eyes and took in the sound of our baby's heart beating. He wasn't in my tummy. I couldn't feel him hiccup, blow bubbles. I couldn't feel him slither and kick. I couldn't rub my belly and feel his likeness beneath my hand. A piece of me was growing outside myself. We had fought so hard to get this far. He was our little champion, persevering. He was right where he needed to be.

Unexpected

I WAS ON our stoop, pulling our luggage out of the house and getting ready to carry it down the stairs to the Uber. Our neighbour walked over to say hi and ask where we were headed. She knew we'd been going through hell trying to give Sid a sibling and didn't know that our surrogate was now almost twenty weeks pregnant. I hadn't felt the need to share just yet.

"Dan has been in London for work and is going to meet Sid and me in Paris," I said. "We fly out tonight. We're going to visit Dan's sister, brother-in-law and niece, who live there."

"Oh, wow," she said. "See? How nice is it to have only one kid? You can jet off to Paris. Maybe it's for the best that you haven't had a second." She might have said it with a lighter touch, but that's how I remember it.

Her words cut me. I don't know why I let them. I would have done anything for a second child. I would agree to never set foot outside Toronto city limits if I could have a second child. I could care less about Paris. It wasn't for the best.

I knew she meant well. She was only trying to help me see the positive. I was being hypersensitive. And besides, little did she know we were slated to have a second. I didn't need anyone's positive spin because I had positive news.

Our trip to Paris was golden. Dan and I savoured our time together as a family of three, knowing—hoping—that in just a few short months, our world would be changed forever. We still hadn't told Sid that she was getting a baby brother. We weren't ready. As much as we were looking forward to Sid touching Kendra's belly and becoming part of the journey, we had decided we would wait until Kendra was about thirty weeks—"good viability," as my family doctor put it. We couldn't bear the thought of telling Sid, who was four and a half years old, that she was going to become a sister, only to take that gift away from her. It was a perk of having our second baby via surrogacy. Mama didn't have a bump that begged questions.

We visited the Eiffel Tower and the Jardin d'Acclimatation, a sweet amusement park right in the city. We visited our niece's school, wandered the streets, set eyes on the *Mona Lisa*, ate too many frites and croissants. We messaged with Kendra, checking in on how she was feeling. On Sundays, we would all check the app to see what fruit or vegetable our baby boy had become that week. I felt jet-lagged—tired and a bit nauseous—but powered through. I jokingly said to Dan that if it weren't physically impossible, I'd think I was pregnant. For many months, we had been actively avoiding getting me pregnant because we couldn't bear the thought of another loss. We didn't use condoms, but he pulled out and we avoided having sex during my fertile window. I kept track of my periods using an app and had just a couple weeks prior logged my day one. It had come about two weeks after Dan and I did a bike race—he rode 150 kilometres, and I did 100 kilometres—and a few days after a cervical biopsy.

I'd had two abnormal Pap smears over the course of a year, so my doctor referred me to an OB for a colposcopy to biopsy my cervix for cancerous cells. After my friend's diagnosis of cervical cancer and after seeing her go through treatment, I was on edge waiting for the results. I was especially nervous because one of the consent forms I had signed at Hannam mentioned cancer. "Fertility medications may be associated with a slight increase in the risk of developing breast, ovarian and uterine (including endometrial) cancers," the form said.

I felt unwell on the plane back to Toronto, light-headed and extremely fatigued. I slept most of the flight, leaving Dan to manage Sid, who was content nodding off and watching shows. When we were gathering our bags at the luggage bay at the airport, I nearly fainted after standing up from a bench too fast. I was convinced something was wrong with me. I prayed it wasn't the c-word. On the drive home from the airport, I was so nauseous that I stuck my head out the car window, thinking I might puke. Once home, Dan unpacked the car and got Sid settled on the couch with a snack. I dry-heaved on our front stoop and then made my way upstairs.

In my mind, there were four possibilities: I had cancer; I was jet-lagged and experiencing the nausea I sometimes get when I'm overtired, plus some motion sickness, which is par for the course for me; I had some unknown ailment or illness; I was pregnant. The latter was implausible for all kinds of reasons. Still, I felt compelled to pee on a stick, just to be absolutely sure. I didn't even tell Dan I was going to take a test. It was silly, a waste. He was downstairs on the phone with the airline because he had accidentally taken someone else's bag home from the airport.

I opened the wrapper with no sense of anticipation. I pulled off the cap. Lowered my leggings. Sat on the toilet. Held the tip of the test midstream. Looked down. Saw the control line turn pink. Put the cap back on. Placed the test on the counter. Finished peeing. Reached for toilet paper. Wiped. Stood to pull up my leggings. Glanced at the test. Lost my breath. *A second pink line.* Two pink lines. *I'm pregnant.*

"Daniel!" I yelled. "I need you to come upstairs! Right now!" I could hear him getting off the phone with the airline. Something about returning the luggage to the airport ASAP.

"What?" he said. "What's wrong?"

I handed him the test.

"What the fuck is this?" he said.

"I know," I responded. "I'm pregnant."

I cupped my hands over my mouth and started laughing as I lowered myself to the floor, kneeling in disbelief.

"Is this a joke?" he said.

"No," I said. "I don't know why I'm laughing. This is insane."

"You're pregnant?" he said.

"I'm pregnant," I said.

"But you just had your period . . ." he said.

"I know," I said.

The only thing I could think of, I explained, was that I mistook the delayed bleeding from the cervical biopsy as my period. The timing lined up. If that wasn't my period, then I was—I paused to do the math—about seven weeks pregnant.

"This is crazy," I said. "But we both know I'll miscarry. It's just a matter of time."

I never thought I'd be back in the Create waiting room, let alone while pregnant. I looked around. I saw myself in every woman there. It hadn't been long since I had been in their shoes. Dan and I sat, sweaty hand in sweaty hand, waiting for my name to be called. I could smell someone's coffee breath, someone else's body odour. I wanted to throw up. The only other time I had been this nauseous while pregnant was in my first trimester with Sid. I would have normally taken the queasiness as a sign that things were progressing well, but after my IVF miscarriage two years prior, I had no confidence my body was telling me the truth.

"Kathryn B?" a technician called out.

"Right here," I said, standing up and gathering my things.

Alone in the exam room, I undressed from the waist down and put on a gown. I sat on the table and waited. Knock-knock. Dan and the technician entered. I scootched my tush to the end of the table, as I had done so many times before. It was time to see if there was a heartbeat.

It was time to see if this was real.

When I tell this part of the story, people say things like "Isn't that how it always happens? You get pregnant when you stop trying," or "I know someone who was about to start IVF but then got pregnant naturally," or "So-and-so's aunt got pregnant right after signing papers to adopt." I have met several women who conceived naturally and carried to term only after "letting go"—only after they had conceded it wasn't happening or found another route to a baby. Sally Rhoads-Heinrich, the head of Surrogacy in Canada Online, said that in her more than two decades of running the agency, she has seen this sort of thing happen a handful of times.

One woman I spoke with, Brooke, had an utterly hellish fertility journey that culminated in two babies born one week apart, one carried by a surrogate (her sister-in-law) and the other conceived naturally and unexpectedly. It took nine embryo transfers to make the baby conceived through IVF. "I say to my husband all the time that we're playing the ultimate game of catch-up," she said, referring to reaching their goal of having two children. "Friends had asked if we were scared to have two like this. No. I am so blessed. We had been dealing with treatment for four years. To me, our family is complete."

Brooke has asked doctors and other medical practitioners why, after all she went through, she would get pregnant so soon after finding out her surrogate was pregnant. As with me, no one could give her a convincing answer.

Why is it that we hear stories of people getting miraculously pregnant when they stop dedicating themselves to the cause, stop obsessing? It's cruel to tell a woman that if she would "just relax," she would have a baby. But is there something to the idea that being at peace could unblock some pathway in the body? Is giving up and moving on some kind of antidote?

"I don't think there's any magic to it," Dr. Taerk, the fertility doctor at Toronto's Pollin said, bursting my bubble. "The chances of getting pregnant is rarely zero percent. If a patient is ovulating, the tubes are open, a uterus is present and there's sperm available, a pregnancy is possible." He has had a few patients who inexplicably conceived naturally after their surrogate either got pregnant or gave birth. Could it have anything to do with the pressure easing? Dr. Taerk was open to the idea but certainly wasn't convinced. "I can't explain it physiologically," he said. "People talk about [the stress hormone] cortisol, but the data hasn't been compelling. If it was, we would be regularly measuring cortisol levels in our patients. If stress prevents pregnancy, we would be out of business."

Dr. Daneshmand had a similar view. If cortisol was the answer, he said, doctors would be prescribing their patients spa treatments and beach holidays. He said stories like mine are simply that—stories. Nothing more than anecdotes. "They don't prove anything," he said. "These types of stories are rare, but they're magnified. They get attention." He made a helpful analogy: Thousands of planes take off every day, but if one crashes, it will make the news. For every unbelievable tale of conception after moving on or finding another way, there are many, many, many, many more stories of people who never got their baby. There are many who are childless not by choice.

How do those people ever let go, fully move on? Do they? Or does the desire for a child burn within them, inextinguishable forevermore? Can the fire at least be tamped down? Coming to terms with not being able to have a child is a form of grief, of mourning a life that can't be had. The grief may be recurring, resurfacing. The healing may not come in a straight line. It likely won't. The death of the dream of becoming a parent can be existential, an identity crisis. It can cost people their relationships, their friendships. And as with other grief, it can be lived with, lived through. Life can and does and will go on.

British journalist Helen Pidd wrote an insightful and revealing piece about her experience going through fertility treatment and coming out the other side without a baby. "I started to seek out others without children, preferring the optimism of the childfree-by-choice community over the grief of those like me," she wrote in a 2023 piece in *The Guardian*. "It has become fashionable to draw a distinction between the childfree and people in my predicament, referred to as 'childless.' Adding 'less' to most words makes them negative: hopeless, meaningless, useless. I personally prefer 'child-free,' not wanting to be defined by what I do not have."

A friend of mine spent years trying to give her son a sibling. She struggled to conceive again, and the one time she did get pregnant, she miscarried. Her husband wasn't dead set on having another child, so he wasn't keen to pursue IVF. She wasn't so sure she was either. She knew how hard IVF could be, with no guarantees. They have continued to try naturally, though she no longer obsessively tracks her cycle. That doesn't mean she doesn't wonder "What if?" during the two-week wait. That doesn't mean she isn't disappointed every time she gets her period. She's in her early forties. She knows the dream of another baby is likely to slip through her fingers. She's not sure when she'll be fully at peace, if ever, but she doesn't feel tortured, she doesn't feel incomplete, she doesn't feel a deep sense of yearning the way she did in years prior.

Another woman I spoke with talked about how her desire for a baby waned as her fertility struggle grinded on and on, year after year. She wondered if this was a matter of time passing, of coming to terms. Or, she wondered, was she becoming less preoccupied with the idea of becoming a mother because her body was moving out of that phase, physically and hormonally? It was an interesting question. Does the biological urge to procreate dissipate with age? Does such a biological urge even exist, or is "baby fever" a social construct? I searched for an answer to this, thinking there would be studies and scientific literature with a definitive explanation. Turns out the question is very much an open one.

Because of our history, Dan and I didn't let ourselves indulge thoughts about a future with three children, two of them a few months apart. We had years before talked about potentially having three children, but as time and treatment wore on, we would always say, "Let's get to two." We didn't want to be greedy. We knew this was Kendra's first and last surrogacy journey, in large part because our child would mark her fourth C-section. I couldn't see us finding another surrogate to carry our third child. I couldn't see a surrogate choosing *us*, out of a massive pool of intended parents, when we already had two kids. I couldn't see us spending the time, money, brainpower or emotional energy when we knew full well that nothing is promised.

The thought of having three kids felt like a tease. I was scared to let myself go there so early in the first trimester. And so I didn't. It was as if I was pregnant but at the same time . . . not. When you've had multiple miscarriages, you inevitably become less and less emotionally invested in each early pregnancy. This was my sixth pregnancy. Staying pregnant wasn't a plausible outcome, so we didn't treat it as one.

For that reason, we didn't immediately tell Kendra about the positive pregnancy test. All of our losses had come before the ten-week mark, so we decided to share our news only if and when we reached at least that point, only if and when we had some modicum of confidence that the pregnancy might be viable. We hated keeping information from her, but we didn't think it made sense to introduce any unnecessary drama or stress, particularly given that questions were looming over the boy she was carrying. Kendra had to have repeated anatomy scans: Technicians were having trouble getting satisfactory imaging of a certain part of the baby's heart. In addition, the baby was not only measuring very small—below the tenth percentile—but his growth between ultrasounds wasn't quite where it should be.

All the while, I was dreading what felt like an inevitable miscarriage. I had been so conditioned to receive bad news about my pregnancies that I couldn't help but believe a loss was a given. I resented the thought of being nauseous and tired for a few weeks only to watch, yet again, as blood spilled out of me into the toilet, scarlet evidence of my body's failure. I had been so happy, so at peace, felt such unbridled joy at the February due date approaching. Couldn't the fertility gods just grant Kendra a straightforward pregnancy and leave me alone?

I put my feet in the stirrups. Cold touch of the probe and ultrasound jelly. Inhale. Insert. Exhale. Wait.

I couldn't see the ultrasound monitor, so I alternated between trying to read the technician's face and sending inquisitive glances at Dan, as if to ask "Can you see anything? Do you know what's going on?" He shrugged and shook his head. More waiting. More silence. I don't remember what exactly happened next, but I think I explained our situation. *Our surrogate is about twenty weeks pregnant;*

this was a natural conception; I've had a lot of losses; we're quite anxious. I think I asked, straight up, "Can you please just tell us if there's a heartbeat?"

The answer was yes. Yes, there was a heartbeat. I was pregnant, measuring seven and a half weeks.

"You're my patient of the day," the technician joked. Dan and I laughed. I looked up at the ceiling, put a hand on my forehead, shook my head in disbelief. Inside the black sac of fluid, there was a whiteish mass of cells, a ghostly figure that looked, at least to my eye, like a tiny baby with a head and torso but no arms or legs. I covered my mouth and cried, completely overcome.

Dan and I met with Dr. Librach to review the results. He came in and read through the papers in our file on his desk. Everything looked normal. Expected due date was May 31, 2023, about three and a half months after Kendra's. We spoke about how uncanny this was, about what a surprise it was. About how when we first met him, we told him we would love to have three kids but didn't want to get ahead of ourselves. "You guys are going from famine to feast," he said.

And then he got down to business.

Because of the extent of the adhesions in my uterus, I was at an increased risk of developing placenta accreta, in which the placenta invades the uterine wall during pregnancy and refuses to detach during labour. If the placenta becomes so embedded in the uterus during pregnancy that some or all of it remains attached, a doctor either has to manually remove it by hand or perform emergency surgery. The condition can, in severe cases, lead to fatal hemorrhaging. The condition is also associated with a higher risk of premature birth, and it may mean bedrest or hospitalization for several weeks or months before delivery.

It was a lot to take in. Were we willing to risk the potential for complications resulting from a possible case of placenta accreta when we already had a baby on the way? Dr. Librach recommended that we speak with an OB specializing in high-risk pregnancies to better understand my chances of developing placenta accreta and how bad it would be if I got it. My stomach was in knots. We had fought for years to give Sid a sibling. We were on track to give her two, and now we were somehow considering the prospect of termination. Were we seriously in a fertility clinic talking about potentially having an abortion? I looked at the sonogram image of the little being growing inside me. I'm pro-choice, make no mistake. This wasn't about the idea of having an abortion. It was about the idea of having an abortion I didn't want.

As surreal, head-spinning and heart-wrenching as it was, we were fortunate to openly have that conversation with our doctor. Just a few months before Dan and I sat in Dr. Librach's office and discussed the risks of proceeding with my pregnancy, the U.S. Supreme Court made the momentous 5–4 decision to overturn Roe v. Wade. The decision had the effect of overruling existing decisions that secured abortion rights, and it gave individual states the freedom to choose whether and under what circumstances they would allow abortion.

The ruling was fresh in my mind as I thought about the question before us in the fall of 2022. I thought of Chrissy Teigen, the model, cookbook author and TV personality who has four children, two of them born five months apart—one via her and the other via her surrogate. Teigen has been open about her harrowing journey, including terminating a non-viable, life-threatening pregnancy at twenty weeks gestation in 2020. At an event in Beverly Hills in September 2022, Teigen was clear that while her baby had no prospect of surviving, and while her life was endangered, this was not a miscarriage. It was an abortion. "An abortion," she said, "to save my life for a baby that had absolutely no chance."

Abortion has been legal in Canada since 1988, when the country's Supreme Court struck down Criminal Code provisions governing the procedure. There are generally no legal requirements regarding parental consent, age limits or waiting periods. If I chose to terminate my pregnancy, it would be relatively straightforward, medically speaking. Dan and I went to the high-risk OB appointment together, when I was about nine weeks along. She was taken by our story. All the loss and now two pregnancies. "Double congratulations," she said. Well, we hoped so, but we weren't sure.

We explained that I had a known case of Asherman's syndrome and that we wanted her advice on whether I should proceed with the pregnancy, given the possibility of placental invasion. The OB couldn't have been more reassuring. There were steps we could take to mitigate the risks, including planning for a C-section, which would allow doctors to manually or surgically remove the placenta, if need be. She also reminded us that we were talking about the *possibility* of me developing placenta accreta, not the *certainty* of it.

Given what we had just heard, we couldn't fathom terminating. The deliberation also felt potentially moot: My body had a propensity for tricking me into thinking everything was fine whilst shutting down pregnancies. My body might well make the decision for us.

We finally got confirmation that Kendra's complete anatomy scan had come back normal. It was a tremendous relief. Our baby boy was still measuring small, toggling somewhere between the third and tenth percentile, but he'd had a couple of reassuring ultrasounds that showed adequate growth between them. We had to let it go and trust that our boy was okay in there. Kendra was our voice of reason, our calm. She would say things like "Guys, he's fine, he's just small. I know he's fine," or "I can feel that he's growing, believe me." Her bump was swelling as she inched closer and closer to the third trimester. I would tear up just looking at her. This beautiful woman doing this beautiful thing.

I wasn't showing yet, at around ten weeks or so, but my pregnancy was progressing too. The genetic testing came back normal. We had also found out the sex. This was getting real. I was starting to feel more relaxed in my body. I was beginning to trust it. It was time to tell Kendra.

We were nervous. We didn't want her to feel like she was any less special or crucial to our journey. I was fearful she would wish she hadn't done this for us—that she hadn't put her body through the needles, the headaches, the fatigue, the carpal tunnel that had developed due to the pregnancy-fuelled pressure on the median nerve in her wrist. I worried she would think that what she was doing had less reason or purpose. I was worried she would think we did this on purpose. She had signed up to be pregnant *for* me, not *with* me. The science may be inconclusive about the direct impact of stress and cortisol on conception, but it was impossible for me to believe that I would have gotten pregnant, let alone stayed pregnant, without the peace and hope she had bestowed upon us.

We wanted to tell her the news in person, so we drove out to Peterborough for our OB appointment and waited for the right moment. The doctor had left the room after doing her exam. Everything looked and sounded good.

"We have something to tell you," I said. "It's kinda wild."

"Oh my God, what is it?" she said. "Oh my God. Are you pregnant?"

We couldn't believe she had guessed it, just like that. She was in shock, processing the two 2023 due dates.

"You're going to be super pregnant and have a newborn," she said, her head spinning.

"I know," I said. "It's crazy."

We hugged her tightly. We put our hands on her belly. We told her this was unexpected. We told her we hoped she knew that this didn't change how we felt about her or the pregnancy she was carrying. She was giving us the gift of two babies.

Two baby boys.

Our loved ones reacted with obvious shock and elation when we told them that I, too, was pregnant. Tears were shed. Laughs were had. There were holy shits and oh my Gods. As my mom put it, we had gone from the sublime to the ridiculous. Dan and I knew we were in for a wild ride, going from one to three children in such a short period of time, but we had been on a torturous path for so long that we felt more than ready, more than able. "It's as if the problems of the past couple of years have become their inverse, and on speed," my sister-in-law wrote me.

It wasn't all sunshine and roses. Understandably, Kendra struggled with the new reality. She's an angel, but she's also human. She felt as though her journey had lost some of its meaning, as if perhaps she should have chosen to help someone with zero chance at natural conception. She worried we may have regretted going down this path with her. She felt like we seemed a bit less invested in her pregnancy, a bit distracted. We had been conscious that my pregnancy would likely shift something inside her and had been doing our best to try to reassure her, but we hadn't done enough or we hadn't done it quite right. Or perhaps there was nothing, really, we could have said or done that would have restored her emotional state to what it was before.

Around this time, we decided to bring Sid in the loop. We considered telling her about Kendra's pregnancy first and waiting until I was further along to tell her about mine. But we thought it would be even more confusing for her if we trickled out news of babies rather than telling her about both at once.

On a Wednesday evening in November 2022, after Sid and I had showered and put on our pyjamas, we sat on the couch with Dan in the family room. I surreptitiously set up my phone to record and then read her the illustrated children's book *What Makes a Baby* by Cory Silverberg. A friend who had children through surrogacy had recommended that I read it to Sid, as it explicitly but age-appropriately explains how babies are made. In gender-neutral terms, it spells out what's required to make a baby: sperm, egg, uterus. We hoped the book would lay the groundwork for our conversation with Sid, because we knew it would be hard for her to wrap her head around the idea that one of her brothers was growing inside me and the other was growing inside someone else. I finished reading the book and turned to face Sid, who was two months shy of her fifth birthday. Her wet hair not yet brushed, she was under Dan's arm, cozy. I set the book down on the table.

Me: "So, we've been waiting for a baby to be born."

Sid: "When?" (Her face lit up with what looked like a knowing smile, though we could tell she wasn't sure if this conversation was going where she thought it was.)

Me: "Mommy's uterus wasn't ready for a long time. Do you remember our friend Kendra? And her family?"

Sid: "Yeah."

Me: "So, Kendra has a baby growing inside her tummy, and that baby was made from Daddy's sperm and Mommy's eggs. So that baby is going to be your baby brother."

Sid: "Cool!" (She sat up, a huge smile on her face, her cheeks suddenly flush. She practically squealed.)

Me: "Isn't that cool? You're getting a baby brother! Are you so excited?"

Sid: "Yeah!" (She buried her face in my lap and giggled, then came in for a hug.)

Me: "We've been so excited to tell you that! So excited . . . He's coming in February, after your birthday. He wants you to have your birthday party, and then he'll come after. Will you help us take care of him?"

Sid: "Yeah!"

Me: "We have something else to tell you. And this is kind of crazy. You know how I told you Mommy's tummy wasn't ready? And Kendra, our friend, did this amazing thing for us by growing our baby inside her tummy? Isn't that amazing and so nice and so kind? She did that beautiful thing for us, because we couldn't do it ourselves. We needed help. But something magic happened, and Mommy's tummy got ready."

(Sid looked up at me with a glint in her eyes, smiling.)

Me: "Mommy has a baby in her tummy too."

Sid: "Now?!"

Me: "Right now."

Sid: "So that means I'll have a cousin and a baby brother?"

Me: "You actually are going to have two baby brothers, because there's a boy in here and a baby boy in Kendra."

Sid: "That's funny."

Me: "So you get to be a big sister!"

Sid: "To two babies!"

Me: "To two babies. You get to be a big sister to two babies."

She shot off the couch and started rattling off all the things we needed to get for her babies—clothes, diapers, toys, stuffies. "Can we go to the store now?" she asked. It was already past her bedtime. We would go the next day, I told her. Her excitement was so pure, so genuine, so palpable. The joy of that November evening put a dent in the trauma we had endured. I was starting to feel like it might be true what they say: Someday, when it's all over, it will be behind you.

—

On a snowy day in December 2022, Sid, Dan and I drove out to Kendra's home. We wanted to take some photos to capture Kendra's pregnancy and our two families intertwined. I wanted to memorialize what she was doing for us, freeze in time her thirty-one-week bump. I planned to frame a photo of her and put together a book documenting her journey. Kendra took Sid's hand and went a few steps further into the snow-covered field behind her home. Sid rubbed Kendra's belly and looked up. Their eyes met, and they smiled. They had by now spent enough time together to feel comfortable.

We were about two months out from Kendra's due date and had started thinking about what day we should book for her planned C-section. We landed on February 10, though we knew the date might be moved up depending on circumstances. The baby was still measuring quite small, possibly a function of some kind of uterine growth restriction, so an earlier delivery may be recommended. In addition, and of great concern, Kendra's blood pressure readings had on a couple of occasions registered on the higher side of normal, giving rise to concerns about pre-eclampsia. If left untreated, pre-eclampsia could lead to serious and potentially fatal complications for Kendra and the baby. Early delivery is often recommended, in addition to medications to lower blood pressure. Thankfully, Kendra's lab work came back normal, without the telltale high levels of protein in her urine. We got her an at-home blood pressure cuff so she could check herself regularly.

Kendra's C-section would happen at the Peterborough hospital, not far from her home. Dan and I had met with a social worker at the hospital, who acts as a liaison to help intended parents and their surrogate prepare for delivery. There are some unique considerations. Because Dan and I wouldn't technically be patients of the hospital, we couldn't be guaranteed a room to stay in after the baby was born. When it came to patient care, Kendra's wishes would come first. Her body, her decisions. In addition, only one support person would be allowed in the operating room during the C-section. As the patient, Kendra would choose whether she wanted me at her side or her husband. If I was going to be in the OR, I knew Kendra would want me to be handed the baby first. She knew how important that was to me. I wasn't particular about much at this point, and I wasn't worried that our baby wouldn't come to know who his mother was, but I wanted our baby, as soon as humanly possible, to smell me, hear my voice, touch my skin, feel my beating heart.

We also needed to think about how and what we would feed the baby. I wouldn't yet be producing breastmilk, so it was a question of whether the baby would get formula or Kendra's breastmilk or a combination of both. Kendra told us she was planning to pump breastmilk for us to give by bottle. She knew that producing breastmilk would help her hormones normalize and her uterus shrink back to size. Giving the baby her breastmilk by bottle was one thing. But what would we do in the wake of delivery when it came to feeding the baby her colostrum, the nutrient-dense, antibody-rich fluid a woman produces before her breastmilk comes in? Would the baby get the so-called liquid gold straight from her nipple, or would Kendra express it so that Dan or I could give it to him by spoon? You might think that I would bristle at the thought of our baby at the breast of another woman, particularly the one who had grown him, but I was open-minded. I knew that babies don't always do what we want them to. If he refused the colostrum by spoon, I thought I would probably be fine with him getting it straight from the source.

I couldn't know how I would feel or what I would do until I was actually in the situation. That was a common theme in our surrogacy journey. I'd had no idea what kind of relationship we would have with Kendra while she was pregnant. I didn't know how it would feel to see someone else's belly full with my baby. In just the same way, I didn't know what it would be like to see Kendra hold our baby, if I would feel insecure at the bond, at the history that already existed between them. I could choose to be envious, or I could choose to be grateful that our son would have someone on this earth who loves him the way she did. No one will have known our son longer than her. She knew him before he would take his first breath.

Dear Life

ON JANUARY 16, 2023, one day before Sid's fifth birthday, I was startled from sleep by the sound of my cellphone ringing. I had started keeping the ringer on, just in case. It was shortly after 6 a.m. Only one person would be trying to reach me that early.

"Kathryn," Kendra said, her voice stern but exhilarated. "My water broke. This is happening."

Her husband at the wheel, she was en route to the hospital. This wasn't a situation where she should stay home until she started having regular, painful contractions. She needed to have a C-section.

We had been waiting nearly four years for this moment, and yet it felt too soon. Kendra was only thirty-five weeks pregnant. A birth at this gestational age is considered premature. We were scared. "Okay," I remember telling her. "It's okay. Dan and I are coming as soon as we can."

It was a Monday, a school day, so we arranged to have Dan's mom drop off Sid at her kindergarten class. We threw some things into a duffle bag—phone chargers, a change of clothes—and grabbed the diaper bag I had just packed a few days prior in case our baby came early. I held Dan's hand as he sped along the highway, headed for Peterborough.

When we got to the hospital, we parked and walked toward the front entrance. As we got closer, I was taken back to this very place, nearly four years before. The pity of the ultrasound technician. The cold damp cement. The loss of *not much of anything.* Our first miscarriage after Sid. What started at the Peterborough hospital would hopefully come full circle there.

We took the elevator to the Labour and Delivery floor. Kendra was there, in bed in a hospital gown, with a fetal monitor wrapped around her belly. Her hair was tossed in a high ponytail. We hugged her and Seb and spoke about how unexpected this was. Kendra had decided that she wanted me in the OR with her. Dan and Seb would be just outside the room, waiting. My memory of this time is at once crystal clear and hazy, a series of lucid moments strung together with a fuzzy thread. Kendra was taken into the OR first, at around 12:45 p.m., to be prepped for surgery. I was called into the room twenty minutes later.

I took a seat at Kendra's shoulders, her body stretched out in front of us with a sheet drawn at her midsection to conceal what would soon be her open womb. C-sections are common and routine, but that doesn't mean they're child's play. The doctor must make multiple incisions deeper and deeper into the body—through skin, fat, fascia, abdominal muscle, connective tissue, the uterus and, finally, the amniotic sac. The bladder and intestines must be moved aside during the procedure. I couldn't believe Kendra had signed up for this. She was nervous but she had done this before.

I could feel my heart racing, my breathing becoming shallow. My nervous system was firing, pent up with years of pining and failing and fighting. My body felt like a shaken soda, about to explode. I kept my hand on her shoulder and kept kissing the top of her head, thanking her for what she was about to do, what she had already done.

I remember the anesthesiologist telling me I could stand up and look over the blue sheet, watch as my baby was pulled from Kendra's body. I wanted to see him emerge into this world. It was almost time to look, the anesthesiologist told me. I stood up, saw a tiny body, alien-like and covered in blood, lifted from Kendra's stomach. A knotted cord wrapped around his neck, a purplish face. I sat down, woozy and prayerful. The nurses and doctors rushed him to a nearby table. I shook and waited for the sound of his primal first cry. There was a flurry of activity. Where was his cry? Cry. Please cry.

And then I heard it.

His scream.

His life.

My baby.

I felt as close to high as one could without the assistance of drugs or delivery hormones. I trembled like a leaf in the wind as tears streamed down my face. I kissed the top of Kendra's head over and over and over, buried my head into the crook of her neck. Lost myself. Someone brought over my baby, let me kiss his head before whisking him away again. I remember saying "Oh my God" and "Thank you" over and over again.

Our fertility odyssey flashed before me. I could smell the clinics, hear the doctors' condolences, feel the needles going into my arms and stomach, taste the tears, feel Dan's body wrapped around mine, vibrating. I felt the weight of it all. And then I felt it floating off me. It was like an exorcism of pain. The sadness and frustration that had been living inside me poured out through a river of tears. The struggle was over. Purged. It was total and utter catharsis. Relief. Release.

I don't remember leaving the OR. My memory goes straight to throwing my arms around Dan in the NICU. "He's here," I cried. "He's here." I embraced Seb, told him I was in awe of his wife, who was in the OR getting stitched up. She had brought us our baby: Oliver Miles Baum, four pounds, ten ounces. He had travelled four years to get to us. He was our eighth embryo transfer. Seven unrealized babies before him. Oliver, and Oliver alone, was destined to be ours.

"It was such a surreal feeling—a combination of relief that he was here, and concern that somehow, even after he was born, something was going to go wrong," Dan said, thinking back. "He came too early and was so small. We had been through so much."

We had been holding our breath for so long that we didn't know how to exhale. It would be several hours before we would get to hold Oliver for the first time. He needed oxygen supplementation and a machine to help the air reach his lungs. He needed a chest X-ray. He needed a nasogastric feeding tube to bring fluids through his nose to his stomach. He needed to rest in an isolette—a micro-environment for premature and ill babies. His tiny chicken-like body was covered in a tangle of white wires, straps, patches and devices. It wasn't until we removed his white hat that we saw how badly his head had been bruised by the forceps the doctor used to remove him. He had no hair to conceal the zigzags and swirls of purplish blood sitting below the surface of his pale skin.

We couldn't pick him up just yet, but we could touch him. His skin was so soft, so warm, his red lips so puckered and kissable. I took his hand between my thumb and my index finger. I wanted to let Oliver know I was there, to let me know he was real. I whispered "I love you, I love you, I love you, I love you, I love you" into his ear. I noticed there was a bit of blood crusted on his lobe. It was Kendra's. There was something divine about it. I left it.

Just before 3 p.m., Dan went to get Kendra from her room down the hall. He wheeled her bed beside Oliver's. Lying there in her blue hospital gown, she placed her hand on the baby she grew. "I just couldn't believe that I had really brought this little baby into the world for someone else," she recalled years later. "I had an immediate love for him but not in a motherly way. He wasn't just someone's cute baby to me, if that makes sense." She explained that while there wasn't a maternal connection, there was "some sort of unexplainable bond that felt sad to part with."

A couple hours later, after Kendra had gone back to her room to rest, the NICU nurses told us Oliver could spend a few minutes outside of his isolette. We could finally hold him. I stripped off my oversized turtleneck sweater, traded it for a blue hospital gown I could leave open in the front, my twenty-one-week bump exposed. I wanted to feel Oliver's skin on mine, devour his scent, feel his warm breath on my body. I had craved this moment in the way I imagine someone lost at sea craves fresh water.

Finally, baby in arms.

And then I felt it.

A kick. And then another.

As I cradled Ollie, his brother was moving inside me.

The next twenty-four hours are a total blur. We barely got to hold Oliver because of all the devices he was hooked up to and because he needed to spend as much time as possible in his isolette in order to make a healthy transition to the real world. We were terrified that something would go wrong. How could we not be? His heart rate decelerated at one point, setting off alarms and sending nurses running over to his NICU bed. He had forgotten to breathe, as preemies apparently sometimes do. His oxygen levels dipped a bit, but they levelled off pretty quickly. We were so very on edge.

All the while, we had a daughter at home in Toronto who came home from school to find her parents weren't there. It was her fifth birthday the following day, and we knew I needed to go back to the city to be with her for the evening and overnight. After having us to herself all those years, it wouldn't send a great message about her brother's arrival if all of a sudden it meant I wasn't there for her special occasions. I was five months pregnant with all the aches, pains and hormones that come along with that. We thought we had done a good job of meeting everyone's needs amid the intensity—our new baby in Peterborough, our daughter in Toronto, Kendra, our unborn child, each other—but I know now that we missed the mark with Kendra.

Although she came to visit Oliver in the NICU the day he was born, she didn't hold him until the following day. I didn't realize this until much later. She had been keeping it to herself for many months. I knew what it was like to give birth to a baby. And while I didn't know what it was like to give birth to someone else's baby, I could have and should have imagined that the desire to hold the child she carried would be compulsive. We had such tunnel vision on Ollie's needs that we didn't appreciate that touching and seeing him in his bed wouldn't satisfy Kendra's immediate desire to hold him.

Kendra asked me if perhaps a "mama bear" instinct had kicked in. Maybe, she wondered, I was subconsciously protective of my relationship with Oliver. I told her I didn't think so—that I think we were overwhelmed and consumed by getting through each minute with a preemie's first day and night in the NICU. I felt terrible that I hadn't made sure she got to hold Ollie, even briefly, the night he was born. I wanted to go back in time and give her that moment. I felt sick that she had to wait until the next day. I thought we had taken such good care of her in the hospital in those first twenty-four hours, but it wasn't the check-ins or the coffees or the soup from her favourite restaurant that she wanted. Like me, she wanted baby in arms.

Certainly, hormones played a role for both of us. For her, the delivery set off a chain reaction that causes oxytocin to surge and progesterone and estrogen to dip. Oxytocin—the so-called love hormone—helps establish a bond with the baby. It works with another hormone, prolactin, to encourage milk production. Kendra told me she had a very strong maternal need to feed Oliver. Not to nurse him, but to nourish him.

I knew from personal experience that hormones can be a real bitch, so I asked her how she was doing one day while we had some quiet time in the NICU. She was holding Ollie and stroking his head. She told me she loved him and that she felt a special bond but that she knew instinctively that he wasn't hers. She was relieved he had arrived safely and joked that she was getting the good part—the snuggles—without the responsibility or stress of a new baby.

Over the course of the sixteen days we spent at the Peterborough NICU, our baby in the care of an incredibly warm and capable team, I was almost unconscious of the reality that I was pregnant. It was like being in two places at once, existing concurrently in two time zones. I was here, and I was there. My brain couldn't compute that I was growing a baby while caring for my newborn. I would catch a glimpse of myself in the mirror or feel a strong kick and would be reminded that there was life inside me, another baby. Our story became lore in the NICU, the nursing team and other parents gushing with questions and congratulations. I felt like I was floating, running on adrenalin and pure joy. I was expecting, living the unexpected.

Because of infectious disease concerns, the NICU had a strict visitors policy. Generally speaking, only parents or social workers were allowed into the unit. No children, which meant Sid couldn't meet Oliver until he came home. Kendra, for her part, was able to freely come and go. She wanted snuggles with Ollie, her "belly buddy," as she called him, and we were happy to oblige.

I remember one time Oliver was crying. I rocked him and patted his tush, stood up and put him over my shoulder, letting his belly rest against my body in the hopes the pressure would soothe his gassy tummy. Kendra was there for a visit, so I passed him over for a little break. I was unexpectedly hit with a fear that he would be pacified by the sound of her voice, her smell, the rhythm of her heartbeat. I was curious if he would immediately recognize her presence. Truth be told, I was relieved when he continued to cry. She had been the one to meet his needs in utero. And even now, she was the one giving him nourishment by way of her plentiful breastmilk. I realized then how much I needed to be his person, as I had been Sid's. I felt no different toward this baby whom I didn't grow, whom I wasn't breastfeeding. I felt the same maternal relief when the bottle of Kendra's breastmilk touched his lips as I did when Sid had been satisfied at my nipple. I felt intensely connected to him. Perhaps the struggle drew us ever so close. I already was his person. I could feel it, and I knew he could too.

I didn't take for granted that I immediately felt such a deep connection. I know this isn't true for all parents, whether they deliver their own babies or arrive at one through surrogacy. It's not uncommon for a parent to need time to develop a bond with their infant, to feel that closeness. Khloé Kardashian spoke candidly about this on her family's reality TV show, *The Kardashians*. She said she felt less of an instant connection with her son born by surrogate than with the daughter she carried herself. "It's a mindfuck," she said. "It's really the weirdest thing." I hadn't known how I would feel, and here I was.

And while we were all digesting the emotional shifts occurring within us, there were also administrative matters to tend to. In addition to the standard paperwork required to register a baby's birth and obtain a birth certificate, we also took the additional steps to establish parentage. Under Ontario law, Dan and I needed to sign statutory declarations asserting that we should be recognized in law as the baby's parents. Kendra also signed a statutory declaration stating that she relinquished any and all entitlement to parentage. Oliver was always ours, but now he was ours under the law.

Incrementally and with time, Ollie learned to take his milk and formula from a bottle. Dan and I took turns going back and forth to Toronto, one of us with each child, rarely overlapping for more than an hour or two in the NICU. And although technically I started maternity leave the day Ollie was born, I was on deadline wrapping up a long-term project slated to run at the end of the month. While Oliver was under ultraviolet lights to treat his jaundice or sleeping in his isolette, I would sit with my computer and deal with edits.

On February 1, 2023, Oliver graduated from the NICU, his isolette decorated with a playful diploma and a card that said "Your NICU nurses will miss you." I put him in his coming-home outfit—the white knitted set Sid had worn when she was discharged from the hospital. At barely five pounds, he was all but swallowed by the car seat. On the drive home to Toronto, in the backseat next to Oliver, I gazed out the window and watched the fields and forests fade behind us. We were "normal" again. We were us. We were living, not reaching. I looked up and met Dan's eyes in the rear-view mirror. He was quietly crying, tears streaming down his cheeks. He had turned on a song we listened to through hard times—Crosby, Stills and Nash's "Helplessly Hoping."

We were through the hope. We were bringing a baby home.

Sid came running through the front door at the end of her school day. She knew her baby brother would be waiting for her. She scurried over to his bassinet, beaming with a smile. "Shhhhhh," she said to us, her finger to her mouth. Oliver was sleeping, so tiny and delicate in a grey muslin swaddle. "Can I touch him?" she asked before gently running her fingers across his head. "Oh my God," she said. "Awwww." She asked to hold him. We got her comfortable on the couch, propped a pillow under her arm, set Oliver in the crook of her elbow. I put my hand on my belly and watched, in awe that this was our life. "Can I touch his little toesies?" she asked.

She was proud to have become a big sister, told strangers on the street about her baby. That's what she called him—her baby. She wanted to help care for him, feed him, get his diapers but, of course, not change them. It was clear from the beginning that she would settle with ease into her role. At age five, she was old enough for us to reason with her just enough. Looking back, I wish I hadn't obsessed so much about the age gap. There was something lovely about the time and space between our children. It only took us the better part of four years and a grand total of approximately $200,000 to get there.

It's customary in the Jewish tradition to hold a brit milah—a circumcision and naming ceremony—for a baby boy on the eighth day of his life. (Exceptions can be made for medical reasons, as was the case with Oliver.) In the days after Oliver was born, we reached out to a mohel, who is trained in the rite of circumcision. We chatted on the phone and told him that, as it happened and against all odds, I was also pregnant. We didn't want him to be shocked when he saw me at the bris. Oliver had been born via surrogate, we explained. We had no idea the implication this context would have, the questions it would elicit about our son's Jewish identity.

In Judaism, a person is Jewish if they're born of a Jewish mother. I was born of a Jewish mother, so am Jewish. Oliver, while genetically mine, wasn't technically "born" of me. He wasn't born of a Jewish woman. The mohel, who is trained in the rite of circumcision, paused upon learning how Oliver came to be. He told us that based on Jewish law, our baby would have to "convert" in front of a rabbi before receiving the rite. Dan and I were gobsmacked. "But he's genetically mine," I said. "Born of," the mohel repeated. No one had said or done anything to this point to suggest to us that Oliver was different from Sid or the boy in my belly. After we hung up the phone, I looked at Dan and said something along the lines of "No way is he 'converting.' He's mine. He's Jewish." It wasn't long before the mohel called us back to say he needn't take the law so literally; Oliver was *of* a Jewish mother. He would perform the ceremony.

At the bris, surrounded by a small group of loved ones, we gave Oliver his Jewish name: Abraham Nissan. Abraham, for my late grandfather, who was a doctor, and Nissan, after the Hebrew word for miracle.

I'm often asked about our relationship with Kendra after she delivered Oliver. The task at hand was complete, the surrogacy journey was over. There was no unfinished mission binding us together anymore, no appointments, no contract. And while the journey is technically over, there's lasting love between us. The tie that binds us hasn't left. He's here now.

"I feel like it's a bond that is unexplainable and unique to those in this situation," Kendra told me. "It's like we are family, connected for life and will never forget each other and our experience."

I look at Oliver most days and think of Kendra. Tears of gratitude and awe come readily. It's not because my bond with him feels different, not because there's something about him or something inside me that serves as a reminder that I didn't carry him. It's because I know he's here because of her, because she made the decision to help us. This makes it natural for me to think of her and be in touch, to plan to see her, to let her know of a milestone—*he smiled, he rolled over, he's sitting up, crawling, walking, talking.* I send her photos and videos of Oliver being Oliver, a dose of cuteness to bring levity and laughter to the sometimes-challenging life she lives, caring for three children and relatives in need, working an emotionally draining job. Life is hard enough, and she chose to make it harder for herself in order to make it easier for us.

Over the Family Day long weekend, a few weeks after we had brought Oliver home from the hospital, we drove to Kendra's with Sid and Oliver for a visit. We felt no obligation to make the trip, no pressure. We wanted to see her and Oliver reunited, to have her children meet the baby their mom carried for another family.

Kendra told us her recovery had been mostly fine—that the phone calls, photos and messages we had been sending uplifted her and kept her feeling connected to us. She did, however, experience some of the symptoms of perinatal mood and anxiety disorder, which used to be referred to as postpartum depression. The disorder is characterized by a number of symptoms, including feelings of sadness, despair, anxiety, as well as sleeplessness and fatigue. If severe and left untreated, it can last many months. It's believed that the hormonal shift that occurs after delivery plays a role, but other factors—such as increased stress, reduced sleep, and a change in responsibilities—are also likely part of the equation. I felt wretched that after all she had done for us, she didn't feel like herself. She felt sad, tired, low. We checked in on her and arranged for meals to be delivered to help alleviate the stress of feeding her family. "I don't think it had anything to do with not having the baby with me," she said, looking back. "But who knows how our bodies work and what underlying emotional effects it has on our mind."

Perinatal mood and anxiety disorder affects somewhere between 10 and 20 percent of pregnant people and new parents. The rate is believed to be far higher, though, due to cases going undiagnosed. The mood disorder doesn't discriminate between mothers and surrogates; it can and does affect gestational carriers. It also doesn't spare intended parents, men included. One woman who had three children by surrogacy told me she recalled feeling low after the birth of her second child. She should have been singularly joyful, she said, but she felt melancholic. After describing her symptoms to her doctor, she was told she was likely experiencing postpartum depression. She reminded the doctor that she had not carried the child, thinking she was protected against such a diagnosis. She was shocked to learn she, too, was susceptible. "I had no idea that was possible," she said.

Roth Edney, the long-time fertility counsellor, said she has encountered more cases of intended parents struggling with perinatal mood and anxiety disorder than surrogates. People who have struggled with infertility are likely predisposed to the disorder by virtue of their often-traumatizing journey. "Surrogacy doesn't cure infertility," she said. "Surrogacy, when it's successful, solves the issue of not having a baby. It doesn't change the years and years and years of trauma. It's not a light switch . . . People who were traumatized, isolated from their friends, bitter, grieving and sad aren't necessarily going to just return to living in the world again, happy as a clam and leaning into being a new parent."

At 2 a.m. on Friday, May 12, 2023, I was stirred from sleep by a tightening feeling across my belly. I was thirty-seven weeks pregnant and had had false contractions in recent days, so I assumed what I was feeling was more Braxton Hicks. But when I stood up to use the washroom and took a few steps, whoosh, a gush of fluid hit the floor. I looked down and saw a small glob of bloody mucous in the puddle at my feet.

"Babe," I said loud enough to wake Dan, my knees shaking. "My water just broke." My water hadn't broken on its own during my labour with Sid. I'd only ever seen it happen in the movies. Ollie's pediatrician had predicted this would happen just a few days prior. She saw me schlepping the diaper bag and the baby in the car seat, while massively pregnant, and said, "Oh you're going to go early, and your water is going to break."

The contractions became more regular as I gathered my belongings for the hospital. By the time I checked in with the nurses, I was four centimetres dilated. As our OB had advised us to do, we told the nurses that I had Asherman's syndrome and was at an increased risk of placenta accreta, potentially requiring emergency surgery. We wanted to make sure this was on their radar. I lay down on a bed and was hooked up to a fetal monitor.

Sometime around 9:45 a.m., the OB on call came by to check on me. He looked concerned. The baby's heart rate was dropping dramatically with the force of my body trying to squeeze him through. I was coached to try different positions, but nothing was working. Our baby wasn't tolerating my internal earthquakes. Something wasn't right.

The OB told us I needed a C-section, ASAP. The team was already wheeling my bed out of the room when they told us that Dan wouldn't be allowed in the OR. We barely connected for a kiss before I was out the door. The nurses held on to either side of the bedrails as they ran me through the halls to the OR, bumping into swinging doors in their haste. I remember one of the OBs taking my hand in hers, locking eyes with me and telling me I was right where I needed to be. In the OR, the nurses and doctors started shouting numbers and instructions. The baby's heartbeat kept dropping. I looked up at the hurried, focused faces above and around me. There were so many. The anesthesiologist made eye contact with me. "I know this is scary," he said. "I know there's a lot of talking, and you don't understand what's going on. Tune it out. Treat it like white noise." The OB told me I was going to be intubated and put under general anesthesia. Words were caught in my throat, but I mustered a nod. I thought to myself, "Please let this baby be okay. Please let me wake up."

And then it all went dark.

Dan was alone in the room I had left him in, left to worry and wonder about his baby and his wife. He put his head in his hands and cried, hoping and praying that we would both be okay. He doesn't recall how long he waited, but after a while, he went and asked the nurses for an update. They brought him to another room and told him to wait some more.

The next thing I knew, I was blinking my eyes open, the room coming into focus. There was Dan, sitting in a chair at my feet. He was holding our baby boy. "Is he okay?" I asked, drowsy, panicked. "What happened? Is he okay?" The cord, Dan told me, had been wrapped around the baby's neck. He had required a machine to help him breathe. Like brother, like brother. The OB told Dan that my placenta had been "sticky," but they were able to remove it from my uterus without having to do a hysterectomy. I was intact. Benjamin Arthur Baum, weighing six pounds, eight ounces, had made it. My last baby in arms. I placed him on my chest and nestled his head under my chin. His skin was pink with life, his intoxicating newborn smell reminiscent of Sid's and Ollie's.

Sid met Ben at the hospital, setting her hand gently atop his head as he lay in his bassinet. "He has more hair than Ollie," she said with a smile. She'd had four months' practice at being a sister. She knew how to touch Ben, how to hold him and be gentle. After a couple of days in the hospital, Ben and I were discharged. We put him in the same white outfit Sid and Ollie had worn home from the hospital. It was Mother's Day. Sid was waiting at home with a sign that said "Welcome home, Ben." Seeing our three kids together that day, Ollie looking impossibly enormous next to his little brother, I felt at peace in a way I'd never understood was possible. I longed for nothing. I needed no one else.

I was desperate to scoop Oliver into my arms, introduce him to his little brother. But for at least six weeks after a C-section, you shouldn't lift anything heavier than about ten pounds. Oliver, now four months, surpassed that threshold. Dan, Sid and our loved ones stepped up to help, given my limitations. We were juggling two babies, after all. Not twins, but . . . twin-ish? Turns out there's a word in the cultural lexicon for this rare but not unprecedented phenomenon: *twiblings*.

With a bit of time, the boys looked similar enough in age that strangers often assume they're twins. I usually let them believe that to be the case, split their age down the middle if asked. But when the mood strikes, I tell strangers our story. I watch as they pull up their sleeves to show me the goosebumps I just gave them. I listen as they tell me that I'm blessed, that I've made their day.

All of our children look similar enough, with their blond hair and blue eyes, but when you look more closely at their features, Ben is pretty much a carbon copy of Sid, of Dan. Oliver—the one child I didn't carry—is the one who looks most like me. Of our three kids, he's also been the baby most attached to me, who cries the most when I leave the room. Make of that what you will. There's something stunning about it all.

We held Ben's bris a few days after coming home from the hospital. It was a larger celebration than the one we'd had for Oliver, our preemie with the underdeveloped lungs. We were now out of flu season and feeling more comfortable being in larger groups. Surrounded by our family and friends, we gave Ben his Hebrew name: Baruch Shia. Baruch, for Dan's father, Bernard, and his grandmother, Blanche. Shia, after Dan's grandfather, Sidney. At the end of the ceremony, Dan and I both shared a few words with our loved ones, captured on video by a friend.

"This feels so surreal to be at this point, given where we've come from," Dan said. "Thank you to everyone who's here, for your support and your love as we've gone through the last four years. People talk about how it takes a village to raise a child. I think, for us, it has also taken a village to make a child—children, I should say. Thank you to Kendra, the surrogate who carried Oliver. Kendra, her husband and their three kids didn't know us when she decided to do this for us. It's the most selfless, generous thing anyone has ever done for us. We're forever indebted to her and her family for what they did.

"And to Kathryn, I think everyone here has a sense for what we've been through over the last four years, and in particular what Kathryn has been through: all the retrievals, the embryo transfers, countless injections and blood draws and ultrasounds, two [911 calls], eleven stitches, three uterine surgeries. It's insane. You are incredibly strong and brave. You've set an amazing example for the rest of our family for what it means to be fearless and courageous and strong. I'm in awe of you and just so thankful. We've been through a lot of ups and downs. There were a lot of downs. It's beautiful to be celebrating the ups with everyone here."

We thought then of Stacey as well. Although she didn't end up carrying for us, she was a central figure in the village that brought us our child. She gave herself to our cause. We wouldn't have made it without her.

When it was my turn to speak, I read a version of the poem "Footprints in the Sand." I'd read it as a teenager and it had stuck with me, coming to mind on several occasions throughout fertility treatment. It's a religious poem about someone walking through life alongside a higher being, together making two sets of footprints in the sand. At the person's darkest times, though, there was only one set of footprints. The person wondered if they'd been abandoned. But they were never alone. It was in those darkest times that the higher being carried them.

"That's how I feel about Dan," I said, out of breath with emotion. "There were times when I just didn't feel like I could keep going. I know I did a lot physically and went through a lot emotionally, but I do believe that these kids are here because he persevered, because he carried me when it was too hard."

I then turned to Sid, who was in Dan's arms, her cheeks blushing with the attention. "Sid, I just want to say that you are the one who got us through so many hard times," I said. "Your little blond curls. I would just sniff them. I'm so proud of the big sister you are and will continue to be. I'm just so grateful for you. We love you so much."

I exhaled. This was what it was like to be living a total fucking miracle. To be out the other side.

EPILOGUE

There Is Mercy

THEY SAY THE days are long and the years are short. The four-month difference between Benjamin and Oliver has shrunk to nearly nothing, though Ben still looks up to his older brother as if he's wiser and knows how the world works. Ollie has taken on the role of Ben's protector, hugging him when he cries, tending to his every need and keeping track of his whereabouts. "Where's brother?" he asks. They look and act like twins, gravitating toward each other no matter who they're with or what they're doing. When they were babies, they had their own language, communicating as only twins can. I sometimes think they believe themselves to be one person.

Sidney has asked us to have more babies because, as she put it to me one night before bed, "they're easy to make." I just about spat out my toothpaste. She hasn't used words to thank us for fighting so hard for her to become a sister. Why would she? But she has shown us, in her laughter, in her joy and in her confidence, that she's grateful for our family, for her baby brothers.

I watch my three children together and I still sometimes feel like I'm floating outside my body. I don't know quite how to describe it except to say it feels as though I'm in the mind's eye of my past self, experiencing my daydreams in three dimensions. It's in the everyday moments that Dan and I catch each other's eye knowingly. Only the two of us know the true depths of what we went through to get here.

I had wondered, before the boys were born, whether I would be an unfathomably anxious mother to them in a way I wasn't with Sid. Would I be terrified all the time of something happening to them, knowing precisely how hard it was to make them? I assumed I would hover and fuss to no end, watch them sleep to make sure they were breathing. I surprised myself. I have been calm. I have been reasonable. I have been joyfully present. It turns out I still have the perspective I earned along the way. It hasn't dissipated, at least not yet. It has been easier for me to move through the chaos of our new life than it would have been had I come by my children easily. I had hoped and wished and fought for years to hear a baby cry in our home. When one does, I can close my eyes and feel bliss. Perspective is the drug that keeps me sane.

Time has passed, but the trauma of what we went through is still there, dormant within me. Though it's not at the surface, it can be easily summoned. I see that sort of access as a gift, not a burden. I can use it to my benefit. So, while I deeply resent the near death by a thousand cuts we lived through, I'm thankful for the emotional fortitude I gained.

I had long thought that the most punishing aspect of the journey had been the inability to satiate a primal desire, the striving for a life just beyond my reach. I had thought it was the relentless bad news that had compelled me to scream into a pillow so no one could hear my guttural release, to pull over to the side of the road so I could pound the steering wheel until my palms hurt.

I realize now that the most punishing aspect of all was the uncertainty—the state of limbo, all the in-between. The quest needed to end, one way or another. We got our wish, so perhaps this is easy for me to say, but I see now that there is value in the quest ending in a decisive way, prayers answered or otherwise. For those who are struggling to start or grow their families, I don't know where the line in the sand should be or what should force your hand to draw it. That's highly personal and circumstantial. I know all too well how easily a line that's supposed to be firm can suddenly become nebulous—how the line can advance, and then advance some more, crossing a boundary set at a more hopeful time. But I think there is mercy in knowing that the struggle will end—two pink lines, baby in arms or not. It can't go on forever. You won't always feel like this. I suppose that's true of all hard things in life. This, too, shall pass.

I still think sometimes of that linen box in my closet. Every now and then, I find myself opening it, leafing through the sonogram images and revisiting the pain of each loss. All these years later—two babies later—it doesn't feel right to throw them away. I'd be lying if I said I hadn't fantasized about lighting those glossy square papers on fire, so I could watch the edges curl, the images turn to ash, the smoke rise. And while there's a part of me that wants to let them go and let the past be the past, there's a bigger part of me that feels sick at the thought of doing anything to erase what we went through. It's the part of me that wants to never forget.

Acknowledgements

THE VILLAGE THAT helped bring us our baby is also to thank for the creation of this book, though there were also many others who contributed to the process and supported me through it.

I want to thank our surrogates, Stacey and Kendra, as well as their families, for trusting me to tell our shared story. They gave me permission to describe—in great and personal detail—the journey we took together. They agreed to be interviewed, taking time out of their busy lives to do yet more for me. They allowed me to mine our text and email exchanges for especially poignant dialogue that helped convey the depth and tenor of our relationship. Without these two selfless women, this book—my family—wouldn't have been possible. Thank you from the bottom of my full heart.

In writing a deeply reported medical memoir, I took the doctor-patient relationship to a different place. Thank you to Dr. Hannam and Dr. Librach for participating in this project, even when it meant answering some difficult questions and treading sensitive ground. Thank you to their staff for providing me with hundreds of pages of medical records and invoices.

This book relied heavily on the expertise of doctors, lawyers, academics, business owners, advocates and others. Some of them are quoted and mentioned by name; others provided insights and information that informed the writing. The long list includes Dr. Tamara Abraham, Dr. Françoise Baylis, Louise Brown, Prof. Stefanie Carsley, Prof. Alana Cattapan, Sara Cohen, Baden Colt, Dr. Said Daneshmand, Carolynn Dubé, Emily Getz, Prof. Vanessa Gruben, Danna Grunberg, Randi Grunberg, Dr. Keith Isaacson, Kelly Jordan, Dr. Arthur Leader, Maureen McTeer, Andrew Meikle, Dr. Dan Nayot, Sally Rhoads-Heinrich, Dara Roth Edney, Dr. Denny Sakkas, Dr. Sony Sierra, Prof. Dave Snow, Leia Swanberg, Dr. Evan Taerk and Cindy Wasser. There were also those who spoke with me on condition of anonymity. Thank you—you know who you are. A heartfelt thanks to reporter Alison Motluk, who has for years so deftly covered the Canadian IVF landscape. Her impressive investigative work has exposed massive gaps in regulation and enforcement. I appreciated her ear and her graciousness.

I'm forever grateful to the fertility patients and surrogates who shared their stories and offered a raw look inside their quests, imparting comfort and wisdom. In being willing to revisit their own treatment and trauma, they helped me make sense of my own. I learned a great deal from my fellow fertility warriors: Alexandra, Brooke, Clare, Emily, Jasmin, Jennifer, Sarah and Tim, as well as all those who shared their stories and asked not to be named. Thank you.

From our very first meeting over coffee, my agent at Cooke-McDermid, Martha Webb, was an unwavering champion. I'm so grateful for her immediate and sustained enthusiasm; without it, I'm not sure I would have taken the leap and crafted a book proposal while in my third trimester and caring for an infant and a five-year-old. Thank you for believing in me and for your sage advice throughout the process.

Thank you to Penguin Random House Canada for giving me the opportunity to write this book and for the work of its stellar team every step of the way. My sincerest thanks in particular to my talented editor, Laura Dosky, for understanding my vision, helping me to refine it and trusting me to bring it to fruition. Laura's keen eye and gut instincts impressed me regularly, particularly on matters of tone and structure. You managed to have a light touch while also having a deep impact—the best kind of editor. Thank you for your patience, attention to detail, thoughtful questions and boundless support. You pulled the best out of me. Thank you also to editor Meredith Pal for taking this project across the finish line and to the outstanding Crissy Boylan, who copy-edited this book and taught me things I didn't know I didn't know.

My colleagues at *The Globe and Mail* were indispensable to this process. These people know the job of reporting and writing, but they also know me. I so appreciated bouncing ideas off them in the newsroom. In particular, my coffee walks with Robyn Doolittle and Renata D'Aliesio kept me sane and motivated. Thank you for your ear and your guidance. It meant the world that you took the time to read my early manuscript and provide invaluable feedback.

I never forgot what *Globe* deputy editor Sinclair Stewart said to me at the outset of this process about what the book could—and probably should—be: an urgent and raw exploration of how and why people fight so hard, just for the chance. It was my north star. Sinc has a way of cutting through the noise and taking care of the reader. His feedback on my manuscript was no different. An enormous thanks to my *Globe* investigations editor, Greg McArthur, who read my manuscript in the earlier days and was a thoughtful sounding board. Thank you also to *Globe* editor-in-chief David Walmsley for our newsroom chats and words of support. They buoyed me.

I managed to find the time and space to write this book because of the family and friends who helped on the home front, carving out windows for me to report and write. Thank you also to Rowena, Maria and Claire. I couldn't have done this without you.

To my girlfriends, for all the listening, all the words of wisdom, all the dinners, walks and phone calls. Thank you in particular to Britt, Pam, Lauren, Liz, Meg, Tiff and Monica for knowing me so well and helping me through my states of overwhelm.

To my parents, Jim and Diane, thank you for fostering my love of writing from a young age and for always supporting me in exploring my passions and taking chances. Thank you for talking through challenges with me and being an endless source of encouragement. Thank you, above all else, for my childhood and the family you nurtured. I have to believe the home you created was key to my desire to become a mother. To my siblings, Adam, Bryce, Mackenzie and Dane, who are the reason I went to the ends of the earth to give Sid a brother or sister. Kenz, thank you for going into the trenches with me and being my safe sounding board. To my mom, Patty, for pushing me to go deeper in exploring the human aspect of a fertility struggle and for encouraging me not to doubt myself—whether through my journey or my writing process. I also appreciate you reminding me to take care of myself when book deadlines collided with work deadlines or upheaval on the home front. To my mother-in-law, Rose, for your endless support and willingness to do anything you can to help make our life easier. To my brothers- and sisters-in-law for lifting me up and being part of my team.

To my children, Sidney, Oliver and Benjamin, for keeping me motivated to report and write, for constantly grounding me in what matters, for finding your path to this world in the ways you did. It was all meant to be. Thank you to Sid for your contagious enthusiasm for "Mom's book" and for asking a thousand questions. I wonder where she gets it from.

This book is as much an ode to my husband as it is a recounting of our shared quest. To Dan, my partner, my comrade in arms, thank you for being open to sharing our story. The vulnerability it required is not lost on me. Thank you for doing whatever it took to make it work for me to find time for interviews, research, writing and edits. Thank you for all the listening, the problem-solving, the hugs and the vote of confidence. This book is my version of a love letter to you and our children.

Glossary

Adhesions: Bands of fibrous scar tissue, which can be dense and thick or filmy and thin.

Aneuploidy: An abnormal number of chromosomes in a cell. Most embryos with aneuploidies are not compatible with life.

Asherman's syndrome: A rare acquired disorder of the uterus characterized by the bonding of scar tissue on the walls of the uterus, which decreases the volume of the uterine cavity. The bonding of uterine scar tissue (intrauterine adhesions) may occur as a result of surgical scraping or cleaning of tissue from the uterine wall, for example through dilation and curettage (D&C), infections of the endometrium or other factors.

Assisted human reproductive technology: All interventions that include in vitro handling of both human eggs and sperm or of embryos for the purpose of reproduction. This includes, but is not limited to, IVF and embryo transfer, intracytoplasmic sperm injection (ICSI), embryo biopsy, pre-implantation genetic testing (PGT), assisted hatching, gamete and embryo cryopreservation or donation, and gestational carrier cycles. Assisted human reproductive technology does not include intrauterine insemination.

Blastocyst: The stage of embryo development that occurs around day five or six after insemination.

Cryopreservation: The process of slow freezing or vitrification to preserve biological material at an extreme low temperature.

Cycle monitoring: The tracking of egg and follicle development through ultrasound and bloodwork that measures hormone levels.

Ectopic pregnancy: A pregnancy outside the uterine cavity. It most often occurs in a fallopian tube. This type of pregnancy cannot progress normally.

Egg retrieval: A common IVF procedure that aspirates ovarian follicles, which may have been stimulated by fertility medications, with the aim of retrieving the eggs.

Embryo: The biological organism resulting from the development of a zygote. This term is used until the end of the eighth week after fertilization, equivalent to ten weeks of gestational age.

Embryo transfer: Placement into the uterus of an embryo at any stage from day one to day seven after fertilization. Embryos from day one to day three can also be transferred into a fallopian tube.

Endometrium: The inner lining of the uterus, also known as the uterine lining.

Euploidy: The condition in which a cell has chromosomes in an exact multiple of the haploid number; in humans, this multiple is normally two. A euploid embryo is a normal embryo.

Fertility: The capacity to establish a clinical pregnancy (as defined by ultrasound visualization).

Fertilization: A sequence of biological processes initiated by entry of a spermatozoon into a mature egg.

Follicle: A fluid-filled sac in the ovary that contains one egg.

Gamete: In humans, a sperm or an egg.

Gestational carrier: A person who carries a pregnancy with an agreement to give the offspring to the intended parent(s). Gametes can originate from the intended parent(s) and/or a third party (or parties). Also known as a surrogate.

Implantation: The attachment and subsequent penetration by a blastocyst into the endometrium of the uterus. This process starts five to seven days after fertilization of the egg, usually resulting in the formation of a gestational sac.

Infertility: A disease characterized by the failure to establish a clinical pregnancy after twelve months of regular, unprotected sexual intercourse or due to an impairment of a person's capacity to reproduce either as an individual or with their partner.

Intended parent: A person who seeks to reproduce with the assistance of a surrogate.

Intracytoplasmic sperm injection (ICSI): An IVF fertilization technique in which a single sperm is injected directly into the egg.

Intrauterine insemination (IUI): A procedure in which laboratory-processed sperm are placed in the uterus to attempt fertilization and implantation.

In vitro fertilization (IVF): A sequence of procedures that involves fertilization of gametes outside the body. Typically, a medical team extracts eggs from the follicles of the patient's ovaries. These eggs are then fertilized by sperm in a laboratory, in the hopes that one or more embryos develops over the course of a few days of incubation. An embryo is then transferred into the uterus. In a successful transfer, the embryo implants in the uterine lining and develops into a pregnancy. The retrieval, fertilization and transfer process can take as little as a few weeks, though an embryo can be frozen and transferred at a later date.

Menstrual cycle: The monthly series of changes the female body goes through to prepare for pregnancy. Each cycle, one of the ovaries releases an egg. Hormonal changes during ovulation get the uterus ready for pregnancy. If the released egg isn't fertilized, the lining of the uterus sheds through the vagina in a period.

Oocyte: The female gamete (egg).

Ovarian hyperstimulation syndrome (OHSS): An exaggerated systemic response to ovarian stimulation characterized by abdominal distention; ovarian enlargement; respiratory, blood flow and metabolic complications, among other symptoms. It may be classified as mild, moderate or severe.

Ovarian reserve: A term generally used to refer to the number and/or quality of eggs, indicating the ability to reproduce. Ovarian reserve can be assessed by any of several means. They include but are not limited to age, number of follicles seen on ultrasound and hormone levels.

Ovarian stimulation: Pharmacological treatment intended to induce the development of ovarian follicles.

Ovulation: The natural process of expulsion of a mature egg from its ovarian follicle.

Pre-implantation genetic testing (PGT): A test performed to analyze the DNA from eggs or embryos to determine genetic abnormalities.

Secondary infertility: A condition where a person who has previously initiated or had a clinical pregnancy is unable to do so again.

Semen: The fluid at ejaculation that contains the cells and secretions originating from the testes and sex accessory glands.

Spermatozoon (sperm): The mature male reproductive cell produced in the testes that has the capacity to fertilize an egg. Its head carries genetic material, a mid-piece produces energy for movement and a long tail propels it.

Spontaneous abortion: The miscarriage of an intrauterine pregnancy prior to twenty completed weeks of gestation (after this point, the loss is referred to as a stillbirth).

Surrogate: A person who carries a pregnancy with an agreement to give the offspring to the intended parent(s). Gametes can originate from the intended parent(s) and/or a third party (or parties). Also known as a gestational carrier.

Traditional gestational carrier: A surrogate who donates their eggs and is the gestational carrier for a pregnancy resulting from fertilization of their eggs. Also known as a traditional surrogate.

Trisomy: An abnormal number of chromosome copies in a cell characterized by the presence of three homologous chromosomes rather than the normal two. Most human embryos with trisomy are incompatible with life.

Zygote: A single cell resulting from fertilization of a mature oocyte by a spermatozoon. After completion of its first cell division, it is an embryo.

A Note on Sources

AS A JOURNALIST, I always strive to ensure my work is fair, accurate and objective. Fair and accurate is easier to achieve than objective, because even the decisions regarding which stories to cover and which people to interview are inherently coloured by the way we view the world and how we move through it.

This book is no different. The way I remember the events and interactions that I chose to describe are just that: events and interactions that I chose to describe. I inevitably recall key moments differently than other people recall them, by virtue of the mechanisms of memory. That doesn't make me unreliable; it makes me human. It also made me all the more motivated to comb through any written documentation relevant to our journey and to conduct interviews with those who came along on this quest with Dan and me. Their perception of what we went through and how we handled it are integral to my understanding of what we went through and how we handled it.

Outside our own circle, I conducted upward of one hundred interviews with fertility patients, lawyers, doctors, surrogates, agency and clinic owners, intended parents, psychologists, social workers and academics. These interviews took place over the phone and in person, some of them lasting several hours. (Only one interview was exclusively conducted over email, with Louise Brown.) In many cases, I spoke with the same source multiple times. I also conducted dozens of fact-checking calls with interviewees to ensure the accuracy and fairness of what I had written. Interviews and fact-checking calls took place between December 2023 and September 2025.

My doctors—Dr. Hannam and Dr. Librach—participated in the reporting process and discussed my medical history with my consent. Our surrogates—Stacey and Kendra—also fully participated in the reporting process and gave their consent for me to publish the personal information contained in this book.

When I quote experts or business owners in the fertility space, I provide their full name and title. For interviews with friends, relatives and fertility patients, I use first name only. Some of these individuals asked to be referred to on a first-name basis, for privacy reasons, and it felt unnecessary and distracting to include their full names, especially since some of these people make only a brief appearance in the book.

In addition to interviews, I pored over court filings and other documents, including some obtained through access-to-information laws. I obtained and reviewed my own medical records from hospitals and fertility clinics, including imaging reports, lab results and clinical notes. I read through hundreds of text messages and more than four thousand emails related to our fertility journey. I also went back to old journal entries and searched through photos and videos. For the most part, any dialogue included is culled from written communications; in a couple cases, I relied on memory and the recollection of others who were present. This book is a work of narrative non-fiction.

The citations, which follow, delineate for readers the provenance of certain facts or figures. Some citations further explore an aspect of the narrative or reporting.

Notes

INTRODUCTION: GREAT EXPECTATIONS

Infertility is typically thought: "Infertility," World Health Organization, https://www.who.int/news-room/fact-sheets/detail/infertility.

A broader diagnosis of infertility: "Definition of Infertility: A Committee Opinion," American Society for Reproductive Medicine, 2023, https://www.asrm.org/practice-guidance/practice-committee-documents/definition-of-infertility/.

One in six people globally: *Infertility Prevalence Estimates, 1990–2021* (World Health Organization, 2023), https://www.who.int/publications/i/item/978920068315.

An estimated one in five women: Surprisingly, there's a lack of conclusive, up-to-date figures on the rate of miscarriage. Studies over the years suggest somewhere in the order of 20 percent of women experience miscarriage. This is supported by anecdotal evidence based on interviews I conducted with doctors. A 2018 practice bulletin on early pregnancy loss, published by an American College of Obstetricians and Gynecologists' committee, lays out some of the estimates, broken down by age range, with additional sources for the figures: https://www.acog.org/clinical/clinical-guidance/practice-bulletin/articles/2018/11/early-pregnancy-loss.

Sperm counts and sperm quality: H. Levine, N. Jørgensen, A. Martino-Andrade, J. Mendiola, D. Weksler-Derri, M. Jolles, R. Pinotti, and S. H. Swan, "Temporal Trends in Sperm Count: A Systematic Review and Meta-Regression Analysis of Samples Collected Globally in the 20th and 21st Centuries," *Human Reproduction Update* 23, no. 6 (November–December, 2017): 646–659, https://doi.org/10.1093/humupd/dmx022.

Secondary infertility: "Infertility," World Health Organization.

In 2025, a single IVF cycle: Canadian estimates are cited by clinics and by advocacy organizations, such as Fertility Matters Canada. The U.S. family-building education platform Inflection has published a city-by-city IVF cost estimate, which can be accessed at https://www.fertilityiq.com/fertilityiq/articles/the-cost-of-ivf-by-city.

Most patients have to do more than one cycle: *CARTR Plus Annual Report 2025*, Canadian Assisted Reproductive Technologies Register, September 2025. In the United States, success rates are available cumulatively as a national figure and on a state-by-state and clinic-by-clinic basis from the CDC. See "Assisted Reproductive Technology (ART) Success Rates" at https://art.cdc.gov/.

The global fertility services market: "Fertility Services Market—Global Opportunity Analysis and Industry Forecast, 2022–2031," Allied Market Research, November 2022, https://www.alliedmarketresearch.com/fertility-services-market.

Miscarriage rates increase: *CARTR Plus Annual Report 2025*. According to the Canadian Assisted Reproductive Technologies Register, the ongoing pregnancy rate among patients using their own eggs to do IVF in 2024 was 36.3 percent for those aged thirty-five and younger. The rate for those aged thirty-five to thirty-seven dipped to 32.8 percent; it dropped to 24.2 percent for those aged thirty-eight to forty and to 13.8 percent for patients aged forty-one to forty-two. Those forty-three and older using their own eggs had an ongoing pregnancy rate of 6.6 percent.

Most people don't go back for them: S. Loreti, E. Darici, J. Nekkebroeck, P. Drakopoulos, L. Van Landuyt, N. De Munck, H. Tournaye, and M. De Vos, "A 10-Year Follow-Up of Reproductive Outcomes in Women Attempting Motherhood After Elective Oocyte Cryopreservation," *Human Reproduction* 39, no. 2 (February 2024): 355–363, https://doi.org/10.1093/humrep/dead267.

OCTOBER 12, 2021

It's 2:47 a.m.: Details from my ER visit are pulled from my personal medical records.

BEFORE

I wasn't tracking my cycle: "Calculating Your Monthly Fertility Window," Johns Hopkins Medicine, https://www.hopkinsmedicine.org/health/wellness-and-prevention/calculating-your-monthly-fertility-window.
Bloodwork to confirm that the pregnancy: "What Are hCG Levels?" American Pregnancy Association, https://americanpregnancy.org/getting-pregnant/hcg-levels/.
***Expecting Better*:** Emily Oster, *Expecting Better: Why the Conventional Pregnancy Wisdom Is Wrong—and What You Really Need to Know* (Penguin Publishing Group, 2014).
Bleeding in early pregnancy is relatively common: E. A. DeVilbiss, A. I. Naimi, S. L. Mumford, N. J. Perkins, L. A. Sjaarda, J. R. Zolton, R. M. Silver, and E. F. Schisterman, "Vaginal Bleeding and Nausea in Early Pregnancy as Predictors of Clinical Pregnancy Loss," *American Journal of Obstetrics & Gynecology* 223, no. 4 (October 2020): P570.E1–570.E14, https://doi.org/10.1016/j.ajog.2020.04.002; "FAQs: Bleeding During Pregnancy," The American College of Obstetricians and Gynecologists, https://www.acog.org/womens-health/faqs/bleeding-during-pregnancy.
I knew from Oster's book: Oster, *Expecting Better.*

SOMETHING FROM NOTHING

Most subchorionic hematomas: "Subchorionic Hematoma," Cleveland Clinic, https://my.clevelandclinic.org/health/symptoms/23511-subchorionic-hematoma.

Genetic issues with the embryo: P. Melo, R. Dhillon-Smith, A. Islam, A. Devall, and A. Coomarasamy, "Genetic Causes of Sporadic and Recurrent Miscarriage," *Fertility and Sterility* 120, no. 5 (November 2023): P940–944, https://doi.org/10.1016/j.fertnstert.2023.08.952.

Those two losses, she explained: S. Sierra, J. Min, J. Saumet, H. Shapiro, C. Sylvestre, J. Roberts, K. Liu, W. Buckett, M. P. Velez, and N. Mahutte, "The Investigation and Management of Recurrent Early Pregnancy Loss: A Canadian Fertility and Andrology Society Clinical Practice Guideline," *Reproductive Biomedicine Online* 50, no. 3 (March 2025): 104456, https://doi.org/10.1016/j.rbmo.2024.104456.

MY ROMAN EMPIRE

hCG to go back down to zero: "Overview: Miscarriage," NHS, https://www.nhs.uk/conditions/miscarriage/.

Doctors recommended waiting: G. A. Tessema, S. E. Håberg, G. Pereira, A. K. Regan, J. Dunne, and M. C. Magnus, "Interpregnancy Interval and Adverse Pregnancy Outcomes Among Pregnancies Following Miscarriages or Induced Abortions in Norway (2008–2016): A Cohort Study," *PLOS Medicine* 19, no. 11 (November 2022): e1004139, https://doi.org/10.1371/journal.pmed.1004129.

Two options to manage the miscarriage: Z. Williams, A. Revelli, C. Cross, and D. de Ziegler, "Natural vs. Medical vs. Surgical Miscarriage Management?," Fertility iQ by Inflection, https://www.fertilityiq.com/fertilityiq/miscarriage/options-for-managing-miscarriage.

Mifegymiso, colloquially known as the abortion pill: Kathryn Blaze Baum, "Health Canada Eases Restrictions on Abortion Pill

Mifegymiso," *The Globe and Mail*, November 7, 2017, https://www.theglobeandmail.com/news/national/health-canada-eases-restrictions-on-abortion-pill-mifegymiso/article36860275/.

Choose to end their pregnancies: Health Canada guidelines say Mifegymiso shouldn't be used in patients with an ectopic pregnancy, which develops in the fallopian tube instead of the uterus. "The use of Mifegymiso could mask a ruptured ectopic pregnancy as the symptoms associated with both may be similar," the 2019 updated guidance reads. Less than 5 percent of pregnancies are ectopic, but the consequences of them can be grave. If not detected early enough, a rupture of a fallopian tube can cause fatal blood loss. An ectopic pregnancy may require surgery to remove the tube and the administration of a chemotherapy drug to stop rapid cell division. Patients who have to go on the chemo drug are generally advised to wait three to six months before trying to conceive again. More info on Mifegymiso can be accessed at "Health Canada Approves Updates to Mifegymiso Prescribing Information: Ultrasound No Longer Mandatory," Health Canada, October 28, 2019, https://www.canada.ca/en/health-canada/services/drugs-health-products/drug-products/fact-sheets/mifegymiso.html.

85 percent successful in clearing a miscarriage: This stat is according to Inflection, a family-building education platform that provides up-to-date information published in collaboration with experts in various fields. In the rest of the cases, tissues remain and surgical intervention is required. Those who benefit from the medication approach, the site says, are "people who want predictability (speed of process and location), [and] people who want to avoid surgery." A D&C is considered 97 percent effective in removing tissues from the uterus. The surgical option, the entry says, is for "people who prefer predictability, people who want the process over with, people who would like to go under local or general anesthesia." Z. Williams, A. Revelli, C. Cross, and D. de Ziegler, "Natural vs. Medical vs. Surgical Miscarriage Management?," Fertility iQ by Inflection, https://www.fertilityiq.com/fertilityiq/miscarriage/options-for-managing-miscarriage.

Thousands of D&Cs are performed: The CDC releases data on abortions in the United States, including those performed via D&C. The figures contained in the CDC's report "Abortion Surveillance—United States, 2022" (https://doi.org/10.15585/mmwr.ss7307a1) were released in 2024 and do not include D&Cs performed to remove retained products of conception in cases of early pregnancy failure or ectopic pregnancy. The report states that in 2022 there were 173,684 reported surgical abortions, a category that includes D&Cs. The CDC does not publish data on D&Cs specifically as it relates to miscarriage management or reasons other than abortion.

Patients who undergo a D&C: A. B. Hooker, M. Lemmers, A. L. Thurkow, M. W. Heymans, B. C. Opmeer, H. A. M. Brölmann, B. W. Mol, and J. A. F. Huirne, "Systematic Review and Meta-analysis of Intrauterine Adhesions After Miscarriage: Prevalence, Risk Factors and Long-Term Reproductive Outcome," *Human Reproductive Update* 20, no. 2 (March–April 2014): 262–278, https://doi.org/10.1093/humupd/dmt045. Asherman's syndrome is underdiagnosed for a number of reasons, including that it may go unrecognized in those who aren't trying to conceive or those who conceive naturally despite having intrauterine adhesions.

Genetic testing report: For those who miscarry at home, whether naturally or with the help of medications, there are two options to test the failed pregnancy for chromosomal abnormalities: an at-home collection kit, which salvages tissues to be sent for testing, and a non-invasive products of conception test, which looks at fetal DNA circulating in the maternal bloodstream before the pregnancy has completely passed.

Triploidy is a rare chromosomal abnormality: "Triploidy," National Organization for Rare Disorders, https://rarediseases.org/rare-diseases/triploidy/.

About a quarter of pregnant women: "What Is Implantation Bleeding?" American Pregnancy Association, https://americanpregnancy.org/pregnancy-symptoms/what-is-implantation-bleeding/; "Implantation Bleeding," Cleveland Clinic, https://my.clevelandclinic.org/health/symptoms/24536-implantation-bleeding.

MOTHER OF ALL INVENTION

At a precise time of the month: A. Aguilar, O. Davis, L. Pal, N. Kaul (Mahajan), D. Adamson, and S. Morin. "Conception: How Pregnancy Happens," Fertility iQ by Inflection, https://www.fertilityiq.com/fertilityiq/fertility-101/what-you-need-to-conceive-get-pregnant; "Conception: How It Works," USCF Health, https://www.ucsfhealth.org/education/conception-how-it-works#:~:text=Sperm%20transport.,to%20grow%20in%20the%20uterus.
News crews from around the world: "The First Test-Tube Baby," *Time*, July 31, 1978, https://time.com/archive/6880038/the-first-test-tube-baby/.
British geneticist Robert J. Berry: C. Nugent, "What It Was Like to Grow Up as the World's First 'Test-Tube Baby,'" *Time,* July 25, 2018, https://time.com/5344145/louise-brown-test-tube-baby/.
"Even if the possibility": This quote, attributed to Cardinal Albino Luciani, was given to a freelance journalist ahead of the 1978 conclave that elected Luciani pope. The quote has been reproduced in several Catholic publications, including in *Crux*, *National Catholic Reporter* and *The Linacre Quarterly.*
Pergonal: Keziah Weir, "The Vatican's Secret Role in the Science of IVF," *Vanity Fair,* April 29, 2024, https://www.vanityfair.com/style/story/pope-secret-history-ivf.
Family Global Compact: "Family Global Compact," Dicasterium pro Laicis Familia et Vita, Pontificcia Academia Scientiarvm Socialivm, May 13, 2023, https://familyglobalcompact.org/wp-content/uploads/2023/12/Family-Global-Compact-ENG_integrale_multimed.pdf

Each year in the United States: The Society for Assisted Reproductive Technology publishes annual national and clinic-specific data on the use of assisted reproductive technology, including IVF. This section is based on data released in April 2025. https://www.asrm.org/news-and-events/asrm-news/press-releasesbulletins/us-ivf-usage-increases-in-2023-leads-to-over-95000-babies-born/.

In Canada, there were: *CARTR Plus Annual Report 2025*, Canadian Assisted Reproductive Technologies Register, September 2025.

Globally, at least twelve million: This figure is from the International Committee for Monitoring Assisted Reproductive Technologies (https://www.icmartivf.org/). The California-based non-profit has recorded a steady increase in fertility cycles since it started collecting the data in 1989.

A typical round of treatment: This section on fertility treatment is heavily based on interviews with fertility doctors and embryologists, including and especially Dr. Tamara Abraham and Dr. Denny Sakkas.

Approximately 70 percent of all fertility cycles: N. Singh, N. Malhotra, R. Mahey, S. Kumari, M. Saini, and Nisha, "Should We Be Offering Intracytoplasmic Sperm Injection to All Couples with Unexplained Infertility: A Cohort Study," *Journal of Human Reproductive Sciences*, https://pmc.ncbi.nlm.nih.gov/articles/PMC12057842/#R4; M. Russo, M. Shin, J. Gale, J. McDowall, and E. Greenblatt, "The Use of ICSI for Non-Male Factor Infertility (NMFI): A Multi-Centre Study," presented at the Canadian Fertility and Andrology Society annual meeting, September 23–25, 2021, https://cfas.ca/_Library/Annual_Meeting_2021/_211-_220.pdf.

The grade is based on several factors: Dr. Denny Sakkas, of Boston IVF, explained to me how embryos tend to be graded. In general, the grade takes into account certain features of the embryo's development. By way of example, an embryo might be deemed a Grade 5AA Day 5 blastocyst. The first number (5) refers to the rate of expansion, which is typically graded on a scale of 3 to 6, with a 6 effectively hatching out of its shell. The higher the number, the better. The first letter (A) refers to the state of the inner mass cells that could become the fetus. This is typically graded as A, B or C, where A is better than C. The tighter the ball of cells, the better. The second letter (A) refers to the state of the trophectoderm that could become the placenta. Again, A is better than C. The more interlocking these cells appear under a microscope, the better. Day 5 refers to the day the embryo developed into a blastocyst.

Patients are choosing the frozen route: The United Kingdom's Human Fertilisation and Embryology Authority, the independent regulator of fertility treatment and research, reported a 41 percent rise in frozen transfers from 2017 to 2021. "Fertility Treatment 2021: Preliminary Trends and Figures," Human Fertilisation and Embryology Authority, June 2023, https://www.hfea.gov.uk/about-us/publications/research-and-data/fertility-treatment-2021-preliminary-trends-and-figures/.

MEDICALLY NECESSARY

"Welcome to the fertility casino": Ron Lieber, "A Baby or Your Money Back: All About Fertility Clinic Package Deals," *The New York Times*, April 14, 2017, https://www.nytimes.com/2017/04/14/your-money/baby-fertility-clinic-package-deals.html.

The survey showed: *Inflection* notes that its data suggest that patients in refund programs are treated more aggressively. The site warns that some clinics incentivize or even require the patient to use multiple embryos per transfer, which increases the chances of a live birth but also increases the chances of twins or triplets. Carrying multiple fetuses is inherently more precarious than a singleton pregnancy, including as it relates to risks of miscarriage, stillbirth and developmental delays. "IVF Refund and Package Programs," Fertility iQ by Inflection, https://www.fertilityiq.com/fertilityiq/articles/ivf-refund-and-package-programs.

No province or territory: Fertility Matters Canada tracks provincial and territorial funding. See https://www.fertilitymatters.ca/learn/funding/provincial-coverage/.

Israel is considered the IVF capital: B. J. Peiper, E. Y. Adashi, A. Penzias, and T. Jain, "Global In Vitro Fertilization Utilization: How Does the United States Compare?," *F&S Reports* 4, no. 3 (September 2023): P326–327, https://doi.org/10.1016/j.xfre.2023.06.005. Israel's fertility rate is among the highest globally, especially as compared to other developed countries, at an estimated 2.94 children per woman in 2023, according to CIA's *The World Factbook* (https://www.cia.gov/the-world-factbook/).

Other European countries: C. Calhaz-Jorge, C. H. De Geyter, M. S. Kupka, C. Wyns, E. Mocanu, T. Motrenko, G. Scaravelli, J. Smeenk, S. Vidakovic, and V. Goossens, "Survey on ART and IUI: Legislation, Regulation, Funding and Registries in European Countries," *Human Reproduction Open* 2020, no. 1 (February 2020): hoz044, https://doi.org/10.1093/hropen/hoz044.

It's abnormal for a patient to emerge victorious: According to the "Preliminary National Summary Report for 2023," published by the Society for Assisted Reproductive Technology, 42.8 percent of women under thirty-five had a live birth after one egg retrieval in 2020. I was thirty-five when I started IVF, putting me in the cohort of women aged thirty-five to thirty-seven, who had a 29.7 percent chance of a successful pregnancy after one round of treatment. If patients want to get a bit more granular in estimating their probability of success, the U.S. Centers for Disease Control offers an online IVF success estimator. The tool takes into account some basic information, including age, weight, height, IVF history, number of prior pregnancies, number of prior births, reason for using IVF and whether the person is using their own or donor eggs. See https://www.cdc.gov/art/ivf-success-estimator/index.html.

A simple AMH blood test: L. M. E. Moolhuijsen and J. A. Visser, "Anti-Müllerian Hormone and Ovarian Reserve: Update on Assessing Ovarian Function," *The Journal of Clinical Endocrinology & Metabolism* 105, no. 11 (November 2020): 3361–3373, https://doi.org/10.1210/clinem/dgaa513.

In an op-ed for *The New York Times*: Nick Loeb, "Sofía Vergara's Ex-Fiancé: Our Frozen Embryos Have a Right to Live," *The New York Times*, Opinion, April 30, 2015, https://www.nytimes.com/2015/04/30/opinion/sofiavergaras-ex-fiance-our-frozen-embryos-have-a-right-to-live.html.

Rapid rise in the number of abandoned embryos: N. Gleicher and A. L. Caplan, "An Alternative Proposal to the Destruction of Abandoned Human Embryos," *Nature Biotechnology* 36 (February 6, 2018): 139–141, https://doi.org/10.1038/nbt.4070.

Alabama Supreme Court: LePage v. The Center for Reproductive Medicine, P.C., Supreme Court of Alabama, SC-2022-0515.

In 2025, a baby was born: D. N. Kupemba, BBC, "'Like a sci-fi movie': US baby born from 30-year-old frozen embryo breaks record," July 31, 2025, https://www.bbc.com/news/articles/c3wne86ex9qo.

An episode of *The Daily*: "The Alabama Ruling That Could Stop Families from Having Kids," *The Daily*, podcast, February 26, 2024, https://www.nytimes.com/2024/02/26/podcasts/the-daily/alabama-embryo-ivf.html.

DAY ONE

120 facilities in Canada: *CARTR Plus Annual Report 2025*, Canadian Assisted Reproductive Technologies Register, September 2025. This passage was also informed by interviews with industry insiders, who have done extensive market research.

Most IVF clinics: P. Patrizio, D. F. Albertini, N. Gleicher, and A. Caplan, "The Changing World of IVF: The Pros and Cons of New Business Models Offering Assisted Reproductive Technologies," *Journal of Assisted Reproduction and Genetics* 39 (January 2022): 305–313, https://pmc.ncbi.nlm.nih.gov/articles/PMC8769942/.

When estradiol is elevated: Practice Committee of the American Society for Reproductive Medicine, "Prevention of Moderate and

Severe Ovarian Hyperstimulation Syndrome: A Guideline," *ASRM Pages* 121, no. 2 (February 2024): P230–245, https://doi.org/10.1016/j.fertnstert.2023.11.013.

Half of the embryos: T. Laguna Rodriguez, M. Serrano Molina, M. D. L. S. Romero Olmedo, M. De Andrés Cara, E. Rico Nieto, M. J. Fernández González, and E. Pomares Toro, "P-253 Clinical Efficacy of PGT-A According to Maternal Age and Embryo Quality in Blastocyst Stage," *Human Reproduction* 38, suppl. 1 (June 2023): dead093.611, https://doi.org/10.1093/humrep/dead093.611.

Increase the rate of live births: This section on aneuploidy and PGT-A testing was based on interviews and numerous studies, but mostly the information was gleaned from the Human Embryology and Fertilisation Authority's extensively researched rating document "Pre-implantation Genetic Testing for Aneuploidy (PGT-A)" (https://www.hfea.gov.uk/treatments/treatment-add-ons/pre-implantation-genetic-testing-for-aneuploidy-pgt-a/).

WHEN IT RAINS

Asherman's syndrome: "Asherman's Syndrome," Cleveland Clinic, https://my.clevelandclinic.org/health/diseases/16561-ashermans-syndrome.

A small percentage of D&Cs: C. Smikle, S. N. S. Yarrarapu, and S. Khetarpal, "Asherman Syndrome," *StatPearls*, July 2023, https://www.ncbi.nlm.nih.gov/books/NBK448088/.

Some clinics exclusively offer ICSI: Aware of the rapid rise in the use of ICSI, the American Society for Reproductive Medicine in 2020 released a report on the fertilization technique. It acknowledged that "the additional cost burden of ICSI for non–male factor indications, where data on improved live-birth outcomes over conventional insemination are limited or absent, must be considered." Basically, if a patient has sperm issues, they should go for ICSI. If not, they can hedge their bets and pay extra for ICSI off the bat, or they can choose to go with IVF and hope they have a good outcome at a slightly lower cost. If eggs fail to fertilize with conventional insemination, they can try "rescue ICSI" to salvage the cycle. "Intracytoplasmic Sperm Injection (ICSI) for Non–Male Factor Indications: A Committee Opinion," American Society for Reproductive Medicine, August 2020, https://www.asrm.org/practice-guidance/practice-committee-documents/intracytoplasmic-sperm-injection-icsi-for-nonmale-factor-indications-a-committee-opinion-2020/.

Two or three embryos: *CARTR Plus Annual Report 2025*, Canadian Assisted Reproductive Technologies Register, September 2025.

THE LONG PAUSE

On March 11, 2020: "WHO Director-General's opening remarks at the media briefing on COVID-19," World Health Organization, March 20, 2020, https://www.who.int/director-general/speeches/detail/who-director-general-s-opening-remarks-at-the-media-briefing-on-covid-19---20-march-2020.

The move was recommended: "CFAS COVID-19 Update #1: March 13th, 2020," Canadian Fertility and Andrology Society, March 13, 2020, https://cfas.ca/CFAS_Communication_on_COVID-19.html#march13.

American Society for Reproductive Medicine: "Patient Management and Clinical Recommendations During the Coronavirus (COVID-19) Pandemic. Update No. 1," American Society for Reproductive Medicine, March 2020, https://www.asrm.org/globalassets/_asrm/practice-guidance/covid-19/patient-management-updates/covidtaskforceupdate1.pdf; "A Statement from ESHRE for Phase 1—Guidance on Fertility Services During Pandemic," European Society of Human Reproduction and Embryology, April 2, 2020, https://www.eshre.eu/Guidelines-and-Legal/Position-statements/COVID19.

The World Health Organization: "WHO Fact Sheet on Human Rights and Health," World Health Organization, December 1, 2023, https://www.who.int/en/news-room/fact-sheets/detail/human-rights-and-health.

United Nations' Universal Declaration of Human Rights: "Universal Declaration of Human Rights (Article 16)," United Nations, December 10, 1948, https://www.un.org/en/about-us/universal-declaration-of-human-rights.

On April 29, 2020: "CFAS COVID-19 Update #5: April 29th, 2020," Canadian Fertility and Andrology Society, April 29, 2020, https://cfas.ca/CFAS_Communication_on_COVID-19.html#april29.

I didn't know this at the time: K. Liu, M. Hartman, and A. Hartman, "Management of Thin Endometrium in Assisted Reproduction: A Clinical Practice Guideline from the Canadian Fertility and Andrology Society (CFAS)," *Reproductive BioMedicine Online* 39, no. 1 (July 2019): P49–62, https://doi.org/10.1016/j.rbmo.2019.02.013.

Get and stay pregnant: J. Zhao, Q. Zhang, and Y. Li, "The Effect of Endometrial Thickness and Pattern Measured by Ultrasonography on Pregnancy Outcomes During IVF-ET Cycles," *Reproductive Biology and Endocrinology* 10 (November 2012): 100, https://doi.org/10.1186/1477-7827-10-100.

A clinical practice guideline: Liu, Hartman, and Hartman, "Management of Thin Endometrium." Studies evaluating supplements such as L-arginine and vitamins C and E have been "small and poorly controlled," according to the Canadian Fertility and Andrology Society guideline. It also said that while a poorly designed randomized control trial on sildenafil (sold under the brand name Viagra, among others) showed an improvement in endometrial thickness, the study failed to detect an improvement in pregnancy rates.

FIRST, DO NO HARM

"If those allegations hold up": Susan Kelleher and Kim Christensen, "Baby Born After Doctor Took Eggs Without Consent," *Orange County Register*, May 19, 1995. (Available at https://www.pulitzer.org/winners/staff-37.)

"I have children": Kimi Yoshino, "UC Irvine Fertility Scandal Isn't Over," *Los Angeles Times*, January 20, 2006, https://www.latimes.com/archives/la-xpm-2006-jan-20-me-uci20-story.html.

In one case in the United States: Neil Vigdor, "'We Had Their Baby, and They Had Our Baby': Couple Sues Over Embryo 'Mix-Up,'" *The New York Times*, November 9, 2021, https://www.nytimes.com/2021/11/09/us/fertility-clinic-embryo-mixup.html.

Ontario fertility doctor Norman Barwin: Dixon et al. v. Barwin, 2021 ONSC.

A class-action lawsuit: "Class Action Against Dr. Norman Barwin," Nelligan Law, https://nelliganlaw.ca/class-actions/dr-barwin/.

"How can the damages": Dixon et al. v. Barwin, 2021 ONSC.

Health Canada inspection records: For parts of the section on the Barwin case, I relied on documents obtained through the federal access-to-information system, including communications between Health Canada and the Ottawa fertility clinic.

In 2012, Dr. Barwin: Jamie Long, "Fertility Doctor Quits Insemination After Sperm Mix-Ups," *CBC News*, January 2013, https://www.cbc.ca/news/canada/ottawa/fertility-doctor-quits-insemination-after-sperm-mix-ups-1.1377898.

The college revoked his medical licence: Ontario (College of Physicians and Surgeons of Ontario) v. Barwin, 2019 ONCPSD 39, "Text of Public Reprimand," June 2019, https://register.cpso.on.ca/File/download.aspx?Entity=cpso_alert&Attribute=cpso_alertdocument&Id=c5b71725-f7f6-eb11-94ef-000d3a09e5b8.

This same woman underwent a D&C: "Form 15B-Finding, Penalty and Costs Order," Ontario Physicians and Surgeons Discipline Tribunal, March 2023.

British Columbia Court of Appeal: Lam v. University of British Columbia, 2015 BCCA.

CooperSurgical: "Class 2 Device Recall Global Medium," U.S. Food and Drug Administration, February 14, 2024, https://www.accessdata.fda.gov/scripts/cdrh/cfdocs/cfres/res.cfm?id=205122.

First piece of legislation: Assisted Human Reproduction Act (S.C. 2004), Government of Canada, https://laws-lois.justice.gc.ca/eng/acts/A-13.4/.

Supreme Court struck down: Attorney General of Canada v. Attorney General of Quebec (SCC), December 2010.

Facilities that process sperm: "Guidance Document—Safety of Sperm and Ova Regulations," Health Canada, December 8, 2021, https://www.canada.ca/en/health-canada/programs/consultation-safety-sperm-ova-regulations/document.html.

Health Canada has an online registry: "Donor Sperm and Ova Inspections," Health Canada, https://drug-inspection-results.canada.ca/dso/en/search.

"In Canada, it's a free-for-all": Dr. Leader pointed to the British regulatory model as the gold standard for oversight in the fertility sector. In the U.K., an arm's-length body of the national health department is responsible for licensing, monitoring and inspecting fertility clinics, as well as taking enforcement action if necessary to suspend or revoke a clinic's licence. Set up in 1990, the authority regulates more than 75,000 cycles annually and holds what it describes as the largest register of fertility data in the world.

Searchable map of the country: "ART Success Rates," CDC, https://www.cdc.gov/art/success-rates/index.html.

Evidence-based treatments: In 2021, the Canadian Fertility and Andrology Society and Choosing Wisely Canada—a clinician-led movement to raise awareness about unnecessary treatments in the health-care space—released a list of the top five treatments and tests physicians and patients should question in fertility medicine. The document notes that the incentive structure in private-pay fertility care opens the door to patients being taken advantage of: "Given the absence of universal public funding for fertility services, there is potential for conflicts of interest when physicians or clinics stand to profit from ordering tests or interventions . . . Furthermore, it is well-established that patients undergoing fertility treatments can experience anxiety and stress, and may be more willing to undertake unproven and costly tests, treatments, and procedures to achieve successful pregnancies." The five add-ons discouraged (in the average fertility case) are: pre-implantation genetic testing for aneuploidy; gonadotropins in doses over 450 units daily for controlled ovarian stimulation in IVF; laser-assisted hatching on fresh embryos; drugs that inhibit natural killer cells, including corticosteroids and intravenous immunoglobulins; and performing sperm DNA fragmentation testing. See C. Jones, L. Hawkins, C. Friedman, J. Hitkari, E. McMahon, and K. Born, "Choosing Wisely Canada: Canadian Fertility and Andrology Society's List of Top Items Physicians and Patients Should Question in Fertility Medicine," *Gynecologic Endocrinology and Reproductive Medicine* 306 (2022): 267–275, https://doi.org/10.1007/s00404-022-06453-z.

In the fall of 2023, the British fertility authority published a paper that rated more than a dozen treatment add-ons that have limited evidence to support their use. The authors attributed the growth in the use of add-ons in the U.K. to several factors, including an intensely competitive market in which approximately 60 percent of treatments are privately funded and the availability of information about add-ons online, which leads patients to have strong views about a particular treatment before they even meet with a doctor. "This combination of patient expectation, market forces and a recasting of the professional and patient relationship in an online information age appears to be driving the supply of, and demand for, treatment add-ons," the statement says. "The Responsible Use of Treatment Add-Ons in Fertility Services: A Consensus Statement," HFEA, October 19, 2023, https://www.hfea.gov.uk/media/kublgcp3/2023-10-19-treatment-add-ons-consensus-statement.pdf.

Artificial womb technology: The U.S. Food and Drug Administration held a workshop in 2023 to discuss the ethical, medical and legal issues raised by artificial womb technology. The attendees spoke about the prevalence of premature birth in the U.S., which can result in fetal death or long-term health issues, depending on the age of gestation and neonatal care at delivery. They pondered the extent to which artificial wombs could extend the life of babies born far too early. "Pediatric Advisory Committee Meeting Announcement," U.S. Food & Drug Administration, September 19–20, 2023, https://www.fda.gov/advisory-committees/advisory-committee-calendar/pediatric-advisory-committee-meeting-announcement-09192023; Philip Hunter, "Exogestation for Treating Premature Births and Congenital Diseases: Artificial Womb Technology Edges Towards First Trials in Humans," *EMBO Reports* 25, no. 1 (January 5, 2024): 17–20, https://pmc.ncbi.nlm.nih.gov/articles/PMC10897319/.

BREAKING

Gestational surrogacy: Kirsty Horsey, "The Future of Surrogacy: A Review of Current Global Trends and National Landscapes," *Reproductive BioMedicine Online* 48, no. 5 (May 2024): 103764, https://doi.org/10.1016/j.rbmo.2023.103764.

Surrogates were involved in 1,306: *CARTR Plus Annual Report 2025*, Canadian Assisted Reproductive Technologies Register, September 2025. The number of embryo transfers using gestational carriers more than tripled over the course of a decade, increasing from 2,649 in 2010 to 9,195 in 2019, according to a 2019 U.S. Centers for Disease Control and Prevention report. Roughly 5 percent of embryo transfers in the United States in 2019 involved a surrogate, the CDC report said. Centers for Disease Control and Prevention, *2019 Assisted Reproductive Technology Fertility Clinic and National Summary Report*, U.S. Department of Health and Human Services, 2021, https://stacks.cdc.gov/view/cdc/114642/cdc_114642_DS1.pdf.

It's illegal to compensate a person: Assisted Human Reproduction Act (S.C. 2004), Government of Canada, https://laws-lois.justice.gc.ca/eng/acts/A-13.4/.

Surrogates' Voices project: The Surrogates' Voices project works to understand surrogacy practices in Canada. The team of researchers includes Karen Busby, Angela Cameron, Stefanie Carsley, Alana Cattapan, Isabel Côté, Alicia Czarnowski, Vanessa Gruben, Marie-Claude Léveillé, Erin Nelson and Pamela White. More information can be found at https://surrogatesvoices.webflow.io/.

Some U.S. states limit surrogacy: "Surrogacy Laws by State," Legal Professional Group, https://connect.asrm.org/lpg/resources/surrogacy-by-state?ssopc=1.

Because my blood type is negative: "The Rh Factor: How It Can Affect Your Pregnancy," The American College of Obstetricians and Gynecologists, https://www.acog.org/womens-health/faqs/the-rh-factor-how-it-can-affect-your-pregnancy.

The risk of miscarriage: I. Riishede, C. Berndt Wulff, C. Kvist Ekelund, A. Pinborg, and A. Tabor, "Risk of Miscarriage in Women Conceiving After Medically Assisted Reproduction with an Ultrasound-Verified Viable Pregnancy at 6–8 Weeks' Gestation," *Reproductive BioMedicine Online* 39, no. 5 (November 2019): P819–826, https://doi.org/10.1016/j.rbmo.2019.06.010.

10 percent of pregnancies: X. Dong, J. Shi, X. Liu, D. Liu, W. Li, X. Zhao, and X. Xue, "Risk Factors Associated with Pregnancy Loss After Single Euploid Blastocysts Transfer," *Frontiers in Endocrinology* 15 (January 2025): 1461088, https://doi.org/10.3389/fendo.2024.1461088.

EYES WIDE SHUT

Guidelines for gestational carrier screening: J. Havelock, K. Liu, S. Levitan, A. Petropanagos, and L. Kahn, "Guidelines for Third Party Reproduction," Canadian Fertility and Andrology Society, April 2016, https://cfas.ca/_Library/clinical_practice_guidelines/Third-Party-Procreation-AMENDED-.pdf.

Even after another surgery: I decided not to include a lot of information on Asherman's syndrome and how to treat it, as the condition is relatively uncommon and may not be relevant to many readers. The Boston doctor who performed my hysteroscopy was Dr. Keith Isaacson, a reproductive endocrinologist and gynecological surgeon renowned for treating Asherman's and who moved his practice to Louisiana in 2024. He told me that ultrasound guidance can help ensure all the tissues are removed and that, philosophically, he prefers suction over sharp tools (though he hasn't seen any studies that prove suction is less likely to cause scar tissue than sharp tools). In all cases, the key to treating Asherman's is to minimize the damage to the uterus. Only the scar tissue should be cut, he said. You never want normal tissue or muscle to be removed, because that additional trauma will create more severe scar tissue than the patient initially had. Dr. Isaacson is passionate in his belief that a thin lining in an Asherman's patient isn't functionally the same as a thin lining in a patient with a normal uterine cavity. He pointed to the findings of a study on the topic, which he co-authored, in the journal *Human Reproduction*. The research found that in Asherman's patients undergoing IVF, endometrial thickness measurements don't appear directly correlated with a successful clinical pregnancy. P. Movilla, J. Wang, T. Chen, B. Morales, J. Wang, A. Williams, H. Reddy, J. Tavcar, M. Loring, S. Morris, and K. Isaacson, "Endometrial Thickness Measurements Among Asherman Syndrome Patients Prior to Embryo Transfer," *Human Reproduction* 35, no. 12 (December 2020): 2746–2754, https://doi.org/10.1093/humrep/deaa273.

2016 article: Alison Motluk, "After Pleading Guilty for Paying Surrogates, Business Is Booming for This Fertility Matchmaker," *The Globe and Mail*, February 28, 2016, https://www.theglobeandmail.com/life/health-and-fitness/health/business-is-booming-for-fertility-matchmaker-leia-swanberg/article28930242/.

Statement of facts in the case against CFC and Swanberg: Agreed statement of facts, R. v. Picard and Canadian Fertility Consulting Ltd.

As Motluk wrote: Alison Motluk, "Waiting Room," *Hazlitt*, August 30, 2023, https://hazlitt.net/longreads/waiting-room-0.

A 2024 lawsuit, for example: Rosa Flores, Emma Tucker, and Sara Weisfeldt, "Nearly 2 Dozen Families Claim Owner of Houston Surrogacy Escrow Company Stole Millions to Fund Lavish Lifestyle," CNN, July 19, 2024, https://www.cnn.com/2024/07/19/us/houston-surrogacy-escrow-company-fraud-scheme-lawsuit.

What expenses are allowed: "Reimbursement Related to Assisted Human Reproduction Regulations SOR/2019-193," Government of Canada, https://laws-lois.justice.gc.ca/eng/regulations/SOR-2019-193/page-1.html.

The Canadian Fertility and Andrology Society: Terry Murray, "Support Grows for Paying Surrogates," *Canadian Medical Association Journal* 189, no. 30 (July 31, 2017): E1004–E1005, https://doi.org/10.1503/cmaj.1095444.

MAYBE, JUST MAYBE

Poor dialogue with clinics: L. Borghi, J. Menichetti, and E. Vegni, "Editorial: Patient-Centered Infertility Care: Current Research and Future Perspectives on Psychosocial, Relational, and Communication Aspects," *Frontiers in Psychology* 12 (June 24, 2021): 712485, https://doi.org/10.3389/fpsyg.2021.712485.

The rematch list, Motluk reported: Alison Motluk, "Waiting Room," *Hazlitt*, August 30, 2023, https://hazlitt.net/longreads/waiting-room-0.

Technology that functions as an incubator: A. Berman, R. Anteby,

O. Efros, E. Klang, and S. Soffer, "Deep Learning for Embryo Evaluation Using Time-Lapse: A Systematic Review of Diagnostic Test Accuracy," *American Journal of Obstetrics and Gynecology* 229, no. 5 (November 2023): 490–501, https://doi.org/10.1016/j.ajog.2023.04.027.

THE MAN

An embryo implants: "The First Trimester," Johns Hopkins Medicine, https://www.hopkinsmedicine.org/health/wellness-and-prevention/the-first-trimester.

Subchorionic hematoma: "Subchorionic Hematoma," Cleveland Clinic, https://my.clevelandclinic.org/health/symptoms/23511-subchorionic-hematoma.

But depending on the size of the SCH: Y. Lou, G. Chen, L. Wang, X. Zhao, and J. Ma, "Association Between First-Trimester Subchorionic Hematoma and Pregnancy Loss Before 20 Weeks of Gestation in Singleton Pregnancies," *Scientific Reports*, December 3, 2024, https://doi.org/10.1038/s41598-024-81759-3.

Sex of an embryo before implantation: Assisted Human Reproduction Act (S.C. 2004), Government of Canada, https://laws-lois.justice.gc.ca/eng/acts/A-13.4/.

In the United States: "Use of Reproductive Technology for Sex Selection for Nonmedical Reasons: An Ethics Committee Opinion," American Society for Reproductive Medicine, April 2022, https://www.asrm.org/practice-guidance/ethics-opinions/use-of-reproductive-technology-for-sex-selection-for-nonmedical-reasons-an-ethics-committee-opinion-2022/.

UNEXPECTED

"Fertility medications may be": "Fertility Drugs and Cancer: A Guideline," American Society for Reproductive Medicine, September

2024, https://www.asrm.org/practice-guidance/practice-committee-documents/fertility-drugs-and-cancer-a-guideline-2024/.

British journalist Helen Pidd: Helen Pidd, "Not Being Able to Have a Baby Was Devastating—Then I Found People Who Embraced a Childfree Life," *The Guardian*, April 22, 2023, https://www.theguardian.com/lifeandstyle/2023/apr/22/not-being-able-to-have-a-baby-was-devastating-then-i-found-people-who-embraced-a-childfree-life.

Adhesions in my uterus: "Obstetric Care Consensus—Placenta Accreta Spectrum," The American College of Obstetricians and Gynecologists, December 2018, https://www.acog.org/clinical/clinical-guidance/obstetric-care-consensus/articles/2018/12/placenta-accreta-spectrum.

Overturn Roe v. Wade: Dobbs v. Jackson Women's Health Organization (2002).

If left untreated, pre-eclampsia: "Preeclampsia," Johns Hopkins Medicine, https://www.hopkinsmedicine.org/health/conditions-and-diseases/preeclampsia.

DEAR LIFE

Oxytocin—the so-called love hormone: "Oxytocin: The Love Hormone," Harvard Health Publishing, https://www.health.harvard.edu/mind-and-mood/oxytocin-the-love-hormone.

Under Ontario law: Children's Law Reform Act, R.S.O. 1990, Ontario, https://www.ontario.ca/laws/statute/90c12.

Perinatal mood and anxiety disorder: "Perinatal Mood and Anxiety Disorders," Centre for Addiction and Mental Health, https://www.camh.ca/en/professionals/treating-conditions-and-disorders/perinatal-mood-and-anxiety-disorders.

GLOSSARY

F. Zegers-Hochschild, G. Adamson, S. Dyer, C. Racowsky, J. de Mouzon, R. Sokol, L. Rienzi, A. Sunde, L. Schmidt, I. Cooke, J. Simpson, and S. van der Poel, "The International Glossary on Fertility and Infertility Care, 2017," *Human Reproduction* 32, no. 9 (September 2017): 1786–1801, https://doi.org/10.1093/humrep/dex234; Fertility IQ by Inflection (https://www.fertilityiq.com/); National Organization for Rare Disorders (https://rarediseases.org/); Mayo Clinic (https://www.mayoclinic.org/).

Index